ALTERNATIVE BREAST IMAGING
FOUR MODEL-BASED APPROACHES

T0180558

THE KLUWER INTERNATIONAL SERIES IN
ENGINEERING AND COMPUTER SCIENCE

ALTERNATIVE BREAST IMAGING
FOUR MODEL-BASED APPROACHES

edited by

Keith D. Paulsen, Ph.D.
Paul M. Meaney, Ph.D.

Thayer School of Engineering
Dartmouth College, Hanover, NH USA

with

Larry C. Gilman, Ph. D.

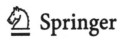 Springer

Keith D. Paulsen, Ph.D. and Paul M. Meaney, Ph.D.
Thayer School of Engineering
Dartmouth College, Hanover, NH USA
Larry C. Gilman, Ph. D.

Library of Congress Cataloging-in-Publication Data

A C.I.P. Catalogue record for this book is available from the
Library of Congress.

ALTERNATIVE BREAST IMAGING
FOUR MODEL-BASED APPROACHES
edited by Keith D. Paulsen, Ph.D. and Paul M. Meaney, Ph.D.
Thayer School of Engineering
Dartmouth College, Hanover, NH USA
with
Larry C. Gilman, Ph. D.

The Kluwer International Series in Engineering and Computer Science
Volume 778

ISBN 978-1-4419-3616-5   e-ISBN 978-0-387-23364-2

Printed on acid-free paper.

© 2010 Springer Science+Business Media, Inc.
All rights reserved. This work may not be translated or copied in whole or
in part without the written permission of the publisher (Springer
Science+Business Media, Inc., 233 Spring Street, New York, NY 10013,
USA), except for brief excerpts in connection with reviews or scholarly
analysis. Use in connection with any form of information storage and
retrieval, electronic adaptation, computer software, or by similar or
dissimilar methodology now know or hereafter developed is forbidden.
The use in this publication of trade names, trademarks, service marks and
similar terms, even if the are not identified as such, is not to be taken as
an expression of opinion as to whether or not they are subject to
proprietary rights.

Printed in the United States of America.

9 8 7 6 5 4 3 2 1

springeronline.com

TABLE OF CONTENTS

CONTRIBUTORS

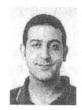 *Hamid Dehghani*, Assistant Professor of Engineering at the Thayer School of Engineering, Dartmouth College, received a B.S. in Biomedical and Bioelectronic Engineering from the University of Salford, UK, in 1994; an M.S. in Medical Physics and Clinical Engineering from Sheffield University, UK, in 1995; and a Ph.D. in Medical Imaging at Sheffield Hallam University, UK, in 1999. For three years he was a research assistant at University College, London, investigating near infrared imaging of the neonatal brain. His research interests include numerical modeling and image reconstruction with applications in both optical and electrical impedance tomography.

 Marvin M. Doyley received a B.S. in Applied physics from Brunel University, UK, in 1994, and a Ph.D. in Biophysics from the University of London in 1999. From 1999 to 2001 he worked on intravascular ultrasonic elastography at the Department of Experimental Echocardiography of the Thoraxcentre, Erasmus University of Rotterdam. In 2001, he joined the Department of Radiology at the Dartmouth-Hitchcock Medical Center to work on magnetic resonance elastographic imaging in breast applications. His research interests include ultrasonic and magnetic resonance imaging, tissue characterization, and inverse problem solution.

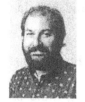 *Alex Hartov*, Associate Professor of Engineering at the Thayer School of Engineering, Dartmouth College, and Associate Professor of Surgery, Dartmouth Medical School, received a B.S. in Electrical Engineering from Northeastern University in 1984, an M.S. in Engineering Sciences from Dartmouth College in 1988, and a Ph.D. in Engineering Sciences from Dartmouth College in 1991. His research interests include biomedical engineering, electrical impedance tomography, image-guided surgery, cryosurgery, ultrasound, control theory, microwave imaging, and tumor hyperthermia.

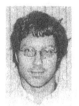
Elijah E. W. Van Houten, Lecturer in Computational Solid Mechanics at the University of Canterbury, Christchurch, New Zealand, received a B.S. in Mechanical Engineering and a B.A. in Music from Tufts University in 1997 and a Ph.D. in Engineering Sciences from Dartmouth College in 2001. His research interests include biomedical engineering, elasticity imaging, reconstructive imaging methods, modeling of coupled fluid–solid systems, and heart-valve dynamics.

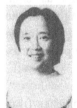
Shudong Jiang received her Ph.D. in optoelectronics from the Tokyo Institute of Technology in 1992. She was a research scientist at the Tokyo Institute of Technology and at Japan Science and Technology Corporation from 1992 to 1998. Her major fields are high-sensitivity optical detection and nano-etric-scale biosample observation and processing. She is currently a research associate at Dartmouth College in the field of near infra-red tomographic imaging of tissue.

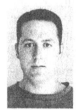
Todd Kerner received a B.S. in physics from Haverford College, Haverford, Pennsylvania, in 1994. He then worked at the Philadelphia Heart Institute as part of a team studying arrhythmias occurring after myocardial infarction. From 1995 to 2003 he was enrolled in the M.D./Ph.D. program at Dartmouth College. He received his Ph.D. in Engineering in 2003 for a thesis involving the design, construction, and testing of an electrical impedance tomography system. From 2003 to 2006 he is a resident in internal medicine at the Dartmouth-Hitchcock Medical Center.

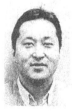
Dun Li received a B.S. in Electrical Light Source Engineering from Fudan University, Shanghai, in 1991; an M.S. in Optoelectronics Engineering from the Shanghai Institute of Technical Physics, the Chinese Academy of Science, Shanghai, in 1997; and a Ph.D. in Biomedical Engineering from Dartmouth College in 2003. He is currently a Research Engineer at GE Medical Systems. His research interests include computational and experimental electromagnetics and biomedical imaging/navigation system design and integration.

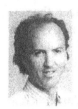

Paul M. Meaney, Associate Professor of Engineering at the Thayer School of Engineering, Dartmouth, received an A.B. in Electrical Engineering and Computer Science from Brown University in 1982, an M.S. in Electrical Engineering from the University of Massachusetts in 1985, and a Ph.D. in Engineering Sciences from Dartmouth College in 1995. His research interests include microwave imaging for biomedical applications, microwave antenna design, ultrasound-based elasticity imaging, and thermal modeling for focused-ultrasound surgery applications.

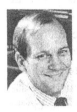

Keith D. Paulsen, Professor of Engineering at the Thayer School of Engineering, Dartmouth College, received a B.S. from Duke University in 1981 and M.S. and Ph.D. degrees from Dartmouth in 1984 and 1986, all in biomedical engineering. He was an assistant professor of electrical and computer engineering at the University of Arizona from 1986 to 1988 and, jointly, an assistant professor in radiation oncology at the University of Arizona Health Sciences Center. He began teaching at Dartmouth College in 1988. A recipient of numerous academic and research awards and fellowships, he has carried out sponsored research for the National Science Foundation, the Whitaker Foundation, and the National Institutes of Health through the National Cancer Institute and the National Institute on Neurological Disorders and Stroke. He has served on numerous national advisory committees for the National Cancer Institute, including membership on the Radiation Study Section and the Diagnostic Imaging Study Section. At the Thayer School of Engineering, Dartmouth College, he teaches biomedical engineering and computational methods for engineering and scientific problems and is head of the Dartmouth Breast Imaging Group.

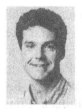

Brian Pogue is Associate Professor of Engineering at the Thayer School of Engineering, Dartmouth College, and holds research scientist positions at Harvard Medical School and Massachusetts General Hospital. He received a B.S. in 1989 and an M.S. in 1991, both in physics, from York University, Toronto, and a Ph.D. in medical physics from McMaster University, Ontario, in 1995. He worked as a research assistant professor at Dartmouth for five years prior to his current position, and has been a scientific review board member for the National Institutes of Health, National Science Foundation, and the U.S. Department of Energy. He is the topical editor for the journal *Optics Letters* and a conference organizer for the Optical Society of America. His current research is on laser-based cancer therapy (photodynamic therapy) and laser-based imaging of hemoglobin in tissue for physiology and tumor characterization. At the Thayer School he teaches electromagnetics, optics, digital electronics, and biomedical imaging.

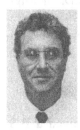 *Steven Poplack* received a B.S. from Stanford University in 1984 and an M.D. from the Boston University School of Medicine in 1988. Today he is Co-Director of the Breast Imaging Center at Dartmouth-Hitchcock Medical Center and an Associate Professor of Radiology and OB-GYN at Dartmouth Medical School. His research interests include breast cancer and breast imaging. He is also the radiology liaison to the New Hampshire Mammography Network (a population-based mammography registry) and the clinical Co–Principle Investigator of the Dartmouth Alternative Breast Imaging Program funded by the National Cancer Institute in 1999. His research interests include breast cancer and breast imaging.

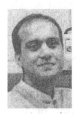 *Nirmal Soni* received a B.E. in Electrical Engineering from M.B.M. Engineering College, Jai Narain Vyas University, Jodhpur, India, in 1999 and an M.Tech. in Biomedical Engineering from the Indian Institute of Technology Bombay, Mumbai, India, in 2001. Since June, 2001 he has been a Ph.D. candidate in Biomedical Engineering at the Thayer School of Engineering, Dartmouth College. His research interests include finite element modeling, electromagnetic simulations, inverse problems, reconstruction algorithms for electrical impedance tomography, and image processing.

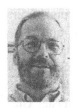 *Tor D. Tosteson,* Associate Professor of Community and Family Medicine (Biostatistics), received a B.A. from the University of North Carolina at Chapel Hill in 1976, an M.S. in Biostatistics from Harvard University in 1980, and a Sc.D. in Biostatistics from Harvard University in 1987. He began his career as a survey statistician at the U.S. Census Bureau. Prior to receiving his doctorate, he was a project statistician at the Kennedy School of Government and the Harvard School of Public Health. In 1987, he became a faculty member of the Channing Laboratory at Harvard Medical School and the Harvard School of Public Health. In 1992 he moved to Dartmouth, where he directed the Biostatistics shared resource of the Norris Cotton Cancer Center until 2002. Currently he is the Biostatistics Director for the Dart-

mouth Multidisciplinary Clinical Research Center and Co-Leader of the Clinical Core of the Dartmouth Alternative Breast Imaging Program. He conducts collaborative research in cancer and musculoskeletal disease and is an active contributor to the statistical literature in the areas of measurement error in nonlinear regression, longitudinal methods, and statistical methodology for image-based clinical research.

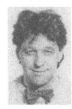 *John Weaver* is Adjunct Associate Professor and Lecturer at the Thayer School of Engineering, Dartmouth College. He obtained a B.S. in Engineering Physics from the University of Arizona in 1977 and a Ph.D. in Biophysics from the University of Virginia in 1983. He is also Associate Professor of Radiology at the Dartmouth Medical School. His research interests include medical imaging, magnetic resonance imaging, image processing, and magnetic resonance elastography.

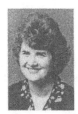 *Wendy A. Wells,* M.D. is a Board Certified surgical pathologist and cytopathologist at the Dartmouth-Hitchcock Medical Center and Associate Professor of Pathology at Dartmouth Medical School. She graduated from St. Thomas's Hospital Medical School, London, in 1982 and completed three years of clinical pathology training at St. George's Hospital, London, before pursuing a residency and fellowship in Anatomic Pathology at the Dartmouth-Hitchcock Medical Center from 1987 to 1992. She received an M.S. in Image Analysis in Histology at the Royal Postgraduate Medical School, Hammersmith Hospital, London, in 1993. Her research interests include prognostic indicators in breast cancer, the reproducibility of breast-cancer pathologic diagnoses, epidemiological studies in early breast cancer, neo-angiogenesis, and morphologic quantification by computer-assisted image processing (including 3D topology/confocal microscopy volume measurements).

PREFACE

Paul M. Meaney, Ph.D.

Medical imaging has been transformed over the past 30 years by the advent of computerized tomography (CT), magnetic resonance imaging (MRI), and various advances in x-ray and ultrasonic techniques. An enabling force behind this progress has been the (so far) exponentially increasing power of computers, which has made it practical to explore fundamentally new approaches. In particular, what our group terms "model-based" modalities—which rely on iterative, convergent numerical modeling to produce an image from data that is related nonlinearly to a target volume—have become increasingly feasible. This book explores our research on four such modalities, particularly with regard to imaging of the breast: (1) MR elastography (MRE), (2) electrical impedance spectroscopy (EIS), (3) microwave imaging spectroscopy (MIS), and (4) near infrared spectroscopic imaging (NIS).

EIS, MIS, and NIS are tomographic. Much as in CT, where an x-ray source and an opposing array of receivers are rotated about a target to acquire attenuation data from many angles of view, these methods illuminate a target with some form of electromagnetic radiation, detect transmitted and scattered radiation, and deduce from these measurements the spatial distribution of some diagnostically significant property or properties in the target. In CT, image reconstruction can be done quickly and accurately by matrix inversion, since the propagation of x-rays through the body is essentially linear, but for the optical and radio frequencies used in EIS, MIS, and NIS propagation is nonlinear, necessitating nonlinear (e.g., model-based) reconstruction algorithms. We employ Gauss-Newton iterative schemes in which recorded data are compared with simulated data derived from an approximate solution of a field equation throughout the image volume. The field equation for each modality is a partial differential equation encapsulating the interaction of the illuminating radiation (e.g., microwaves) with some tissue property of interest (e.g., conductivity). The property distribution is estimated initially; the field equation is then solved approximately over the image space, using the estimated property distribution and the known illumination pattern as inputs to a finite element method; and finally, the simulated data are compared to the real data. If the simulated data and the real data are too dissimilar, the model property distribution is updated (by means that will be described in detail later in this book) and the field equation re-solved. This process is repeated until measurement agrees satisfactorily with model output. Solving the field equation and updating the model property distribution is computation-intensive because it requires the inversion of large matrices.

MRE, unlike the other three modalities, is not a tomographic approach. However, its goal—reconstruction of tissue elastic properties—also requires the solution of a nonlinear problem, and is also achieved by a model-based Gauss-Newton iterative method.

All our solution methods are nonlinear, but earlier attempts to utilize microwave, near infrared, and electrical impedance approaches made use of linear approximations. Although these proved inadequate, the ever-increasing availability of computing power may make some such approach feasible again.

Imaging for the detection of breast cancer is a particularly interesting and relevant application of the four imaging modalities discussed in this book. Breast cancer is an extremely common health problem for women; the National Cancer Institute estimates that one in eight US women will develop breast cancer at least once in her lifetime. Yet the efficacy of the standard (and notoriously uncomfortable) early-detection test, the x-ray mammogram, has been disputed of late, especially for younger women. Conditions are thus ripe for the development of affordable techniques that replace or complement the mammogram. The breast is both anatomically accessible and small enough that the computing power required to model it is affordable.

Chapter 1 introduces the present state of breast imaging and discusses how our alternative modalities can contribute to the field. Chapter 2 looks at the computational common ground shared by all four modalities. Chapters 2 through 10 are devoted to the four modalities, which each modality being discussed first in a theory chapter and then in an implementation-and-results chapter. The eleventh and final chapter discusses statistical methods for image analysis in the context of these four alternative imaging modalities.

Acknowledgements

The editors would like to thank Shireen Geimer of the Thayer School of Engineering, Dartmouth College, for her patient and skillful efforts in preparing several of the figures in this book.

This work has been supported by NIH/NCI grant number PO1-CA80139.

Chapter 1

FOUR ALTERNATIVE BREAST IMAGING MODALITIES

Steven Poplack, M.D., Ph.D., Wendy Wells, M.D., M.S., and Keith Paulsen, Ph.D.

1   INTRODUCTION

1.1   Breast Cancer

In the United States, breast cancer is the most common non-skin malignancy in women and the second leading cause of female cancer mortality. Approximately 180,000 new cases of invasive breast cancer, resulting in over 40,000 deaths, are diagnosed annually. Age-adjusted incidence has remained approximately constant since a notable increase from the mid 1970s to the late 1980s, while mortality, after having remained constant for at least 40 years, has been declining slowly since 1990 (i.e., from $\sim 22\%$ in 1990 to $\sim 18\%$ in 2000) [1, 2]. Approximately one in every eight US women is diagnosed with breast cancer by the age of 90, for an absolute lifetime risk of 14.4% [2]. Breast cancer also occurs in men, but accounts for less than one percent of male malignancies.

The benefits of breast-cancer screening by existing methods, especially for younger women, are controversial, but most experts agree that mammography screening benefits women 50–69 years old [3–5]. Meta-analyses of randomized-control trials of mammography screening show a 25–30% reduction in breast cancer mortality for women over 50, and a smaller, more equivocal effect in women aged 40–49 [6]. Regarding breast cancer screening with clinical breast examination (CBE), the US Preventive Service Task

Force concluded that the "evidence is insufficient to recommend for or against routine CBE alone . . . [or] teaching or performing routine breast self-examination" [7].

Screening might produce greater benefits if it were more sensitive and specific. However, the standard screening technology—x-ray screen-film mammogram—has many unsatisfactory features, as reviewed below. Therefore, a wide variety of new technologies, including alternative imaging modalities, improvements in x-ray mammography, and novel biological assays, are being investigated (and in some cases deployed) in hopes of improving early-detection rates.

1.2   Mammography and the Rationale for Alternatives

In the US, mammography is currently the most effective method of detecting asymptomatic breast cancer. Its use for screening has been widely promoted by the National Cancer Institute and other organizations. Screening is also the primary role foreseen for most of the alternative imaging modalities now being developed. The potential usefulness of alternative imaging is not, however, restricted to screening; it may also contribute to the characterization of breast abnormalities detected by mammography and other means, including breast self-examination and CBE.

Despite its recognized value in detecting and characterizing breast disease, mammography has important limitations. First, its false-negative rate ranges from 4% to 34%, depending on the definition of a false negative and on the length of follow-up after a "normal" mammogram [8]. Second, screening mammography is less sensitive in women with radiographically dense breast tissue [9]. This is of particular concern because the amount of fibroglandular tissue may represent an independent risk factor for developing breast cancer [10]. Third, screening mammography also suffers from a high false-positive rate: on average, 75% of breast biopsies prompted by a "suspicious" mammographic abnormality prove benign [2]. Mammography's other drawbacks include discomfort due to breast compression, variability in radiological interpretation, and a slight risk of inducing cancer due to the ionizing radiation exposure.

Given these deficits, development of imaging modalities or genetic-marker techniques that would enhance, complement, or replace mammography has been a priority. Enhancements of screen-film mammography have included full-field digital mammography and computer-aided detection of abnormalities. Some of the alternative modalities under investigation are ultrasound (including compound, three-dimensional, Doppler, and harmonic variants), magnetic resonance imaging (MRI), elastography, scintimammography, positron emission tomography, and thermography [2].

Some alternative imaging methods do not yet achieve the high-resolution structural imaging offered by conventional mammography. While this would be desirable, there are good reasons for trading some spatial resolution for other information. In particular, providing the radiologist with alternative tools for evaluating patient populations not well-served by mammography and expanding the diagnostic information available to the radiologist in clinically suspicious cases are important goals not dependent on high spatial resolution as such. For example, imaging methods that are sensitive to functional malignant features such as angiogenesis could be exploited in an adjunctive role to improve the specificity of mammographic diagnosis. In addition, x-ray mammography has been repeatably found not to detect 10–30% of cancers greater than 5 mm in diameter, largely due to its relatively poor soft-tissue contrast [11]. This is particularly true for radiologically dense breasts, which are more common in younger women. Spatial resolution may thus not be the limiting factor for detecting certain mammographic abnormalities, and so should not be the overriding concern in the development of alternatives to current breast-imaging technologies.

Since 1999 a group of engineers and physicians at Dartmouth College has been conducting a research program dedicated to the development of alternative breast-cancer imaging technologies. We believe that the four alternative modalities we are investigating—magnetic resonance elastography (MRE), electrical impedance spectroscopy (EIS), microwave imaging spectroscopy (MIS), and near infrared spectroscopic imaging (NIS), all discussed in detail in this book—have the potential to increase the frequency and accuracy with which breast cancer can be detected and diagnosed and to improve the staging and monitoring of disease progression/regression during treatment and follow-up periods of clinical care.

Our program combines technology development with clinical studies designed to establish that MRE, EIS, MIS, and NIS have the potential to contribute, either alone or in combination, to breast imaging for risk assessment, early detection, differential diagnosis, treatment prognosis, and therapy monitoring. We have demonstrated the clinical feasibility of these imaging technologies for breast imaging by initiating their clinical evaluation in a common cohort of women with normal and abnormal breasts as defined by screening mammography and subsequently verified (for abnormal breasts) by biopsy. In the next few years we expect to generate enough evidence to estimate the likely role of these breast-imaging alternatives for differential diagnosis, treatment prognosis, and therapy monitoring. With greater sophistication, the technologies themselves will become increasingly viable choices for risk assessment and early detection. Indeed, a 1998 consensus report by the National Cancer Institute blue-ribbon panel on the future of breast cancer research (*Priorities for Breast Cancer Research*, 1998) explicitly cited MRE, EIS, MIS, and NIS as promising avenues for advancing the detection and diagnosis of breast disease. These modalities have been rendered feasible by the recent explosion in low-cost computational power. They do not use ionizing radiation, do not require painful levels of breast compression, are not likely to be limited by radiographically dense breast composition (i.e, decreased sensitivity in the setting of dense breasts), and should provide quantitative data that can reduce the interpretive variability associated with mammography.

In the following sections, the physical bases of MRE, EIS, MIS, and NIS are outlined, along with the electrical and mechanical properties of normal and abnormal breast tissue that enable these modalities to discriminate between healthy and abnormal tissues. A detailed review then follows of our assessment of microvasculature and tissue-type interfaces in breast tissues having normal histology, fibrocystic disease, fibroadenomas, and invasive carcinomas. This study shows how electromechanical tissue properties can correlate with biological characteristics. We conclude by describing some of our near-term goals.

2   FOUR ALTERNATIVE MODALITIES

All four of the modalities being investigated by our group work by iteratively optimizing a two- or three-dimensional finite element (FE) model of specific material properties throughout some portion of the breast. An optimization algorithm compares actual measurements made outside the breast—light intensities, electromagnetic (EM) fields, or mechanical displacements—to data predicted using the FE model. The model is then iteratively adjusted to make its predictions approximately match observation, and the property distribution corresponding to the best available convergence is used to generate an image. It is because of FE modeling's essential role in this process that we refer to all four techniques as *model-based* alternative breast-imaging modalities.

Below, we briefly indicate the physical basis of each imaging modality. We then describe how we integrate our research on all four modalities into a single initiative centered on two shared-resource "cores," one clinical and one computational.

2.1   Magnetic Resonance Elastography (MRE)

In this technique, mechanical vibrations are applied to the breast's surface that propagate through the breast as a three-dimensional, time-harmonic spatial displacement field varying locally with the mechanical properties of each tissue region. Magnetic resonance (MR) techniques are used to image this displacement field. These data are used to optimize an FE model of the breast's three-dimensional mechanical property distribution by iteratively refining an initial estimate of that distribution until the model predicts the observed displacements as closely as possible. MRE is distinguished from the other three methods discussed in this book by the fact that a very large, three-dimensional data set is supplied to its FE modeling algorithm. This mandates special "subzone" techniques to reduce the computational challenge, as discussed in Chapter 3. MRE is also the only nontomographic technique in this set of alternative modalities.

The principal hypothesis underpinning our MRE project is that the mechanical properties of breast tissue provide unique information for the detection, characterization, and monitoring of pathology. There is much evidence to suggest that tissue hardness is strongly associated with cancer. The effectiveness of clinical palpation for hard tissue in discovering larger tumors is well-established; in the Breast Cancer Demonstration Project, approximately one-third of malignancies were discovered by physical examination rather than by x-ray mammography [12]. Although little quantitative work has appeared on the mechanical properties or behavior of breast tissue, measurements of the sonoelasticity of masses in rodent prostatectomy specimens have shown good correlations with elasticity [13–15].

As detailed in Chapter 4, our MRE team has recovered images based on time-harmonic, steady-state mechanical wave generation, MR measurement, and numerical inversion to form images of mechanical properties at or near the acquisition resolution of MRI. Further, a number of clinical exams have been completed that have demonstrated feasibility, provided preliminary estimates of the elastic properties of the normal breast, and highlighted areas where further investigation is warranted.

2.2   Electrical Impedance Spectroscopy (EIS)

EIS passes small AC currents through the pendant breast by means of a ring of electrodes placed in contact with the skin. Magnitude and phase measurements of both voltage and current are made simultaneously at all electrodes.

The observed patterns of voltage and current are a function both of the signals applied and of the interior structure of the breast. EIS seeks to optimize an FE model of the spatial distribution of conductivity and permittivity in the breast's interior, using the applied signals as known inputs and the observed signals as known outputs. EIS is referred to as electrical impedance *spectroscopy* because AC currents can be applied to the breast at a wide range of frequencies.

In the frequency range of interest for this modality, the so-called β dispersion is sensitive to cellular morphology and tissue microarchitecture, particularly membrane structures (both intra- and extracellular). At the low end of the spectrum, charging and discharging of membranes occurs, which introduces capacitance and forces electric current to pass through the extracellular medium. As frequency is increased, cellular capacitive reactance decreases, which causes an increase in current flow through the intracellular space. This makes higher-frequency signals more sensitive to intracellular influences. Also at higher frequencies, dipolar reorientation of proteins and tissue organelles can occur. Hence, the β dispersion electrical-property spectrum contains information about both the extra- and intracellular environments.

A study by Cuzick et al. [16] supports this view. The authors measured the electrical depolarization index of breasts *in vivo* for 661 women scheduled for open biopsy. Comparison of abnormalities detected from the electrical depolarization data to biopsy results yielded 70% specificity at 80% sensitivity and 55% specificity at 90% sensitivity for palpable masses. The authors hypothesize that the measured effect results from a loss of transepithelial potential during the carcinogenesis of normally polarized epithelial cells, and further surmise that abnormal proliferation extending around the borders of the malignancy into the surrounding regions of the affected site (which has been shown to occur in breast and other epithelial cancers) causes the electrical differences sensed at the surface. If these intrinsic electrical polarization-depolarization phenomena do occur, they will perturb the actively induced electric fields associated with EIS imaging and may produce a detectable, larger-than-tumor signature.

Further, there are significant differences between the electrical impedances of histologically-confirmed diseased breast tissue and normal breast [17–20]. These impedance heterogeneities within and around a tumor can be discriminated with EIS. Further, the dispersion characteristics of normal and cancerous tissues differ. This last fact is of particular interest; it means that it may be possible to create a clinical tool that spatially resolves spectroscopic information in such a way as to distinguish tumor from normal tissue.

The goal of our EIS team has been to develop an ultrafast, multidimensional (i.e., spatio-spectral) EIS imaging system complete with data acquisition electronics, breast positioning interface, and exam-control and image-reconstruction software. We have constructed three generations of such systems, the first of which has been operational for the majority of exam sessions described in Ch. 6 of this book and the latest of which represents a large step forward in capability and speed and is now operational for clinical use. This advanced instrument is a considerable asset in addressing fundamental questions surrounding the potential role of EIS in breast-imaging applications. It has yet to be optimized for clinical use from both the hardware and software perspectives (see Ch. 6).

2.3   Microwave Imaging Spectroscopy (MIS)

Like EIS, MIS interrogates the breast using EM fields. It differs in using much higher frequencies (300–3000 MHz). In this range it is appropriate to treat EM phenomena in the breast in terms of wave propagation rather than voltages and currents. The technologies and mathematics used in EIS and MIS are, therefore, somewhat divergent, despite the fact the both exploit EM interactions in tissue.

Like EIS and NIS, MIS surrounds the breast with a circular array of transducers. In this case, these are antennas capable of acting either as transmitters or receivers. Unlike the transducers used in EIS and NIS, these antennas are not in direct contact with the breast but are coupled to it through a liquid medium (i.e., the breast is pendant in a liquid-filled tank). Sinusoidal microwave radiation at a fixed frequency is emitted by one antenna and measured at the other antennas. Each antenna takes its turn as the transmitter until the entire array has been so utilized. A wide range of frequencies may be employed, hence the term "microwave imaging *spectroscopy*." As in the other modalities, an FE model of either a two-dimensional slice or a three-dimensional subvolume of the breast is iteratively adjusted so that the magnitude and phase measurements predicted using the transmitted waveforms as known inputs converge as closely as possible with those actually observed. The breast properties imaged are permittivity and conductivity, as in EIS, but because of the disjoint frequency ranges employed these properties may serve as proxies for different physiological variables in the two techniques.

Electromagnetic fields interact with tissues through three basic mechanisms: (1) the displacement of conduction (free) electrons and ions in tissue as a result of the force exerted on them by the applied EM field; (2) polarization of atoms and molecules to produce dipoles; and (3) orientation of permanently dipolar molecules in the direction of the applied field. The number of free electrons and ions that are available to create a conduction current within the tissue in response to an applied field is proportional to the tissue's intrinsic electrical conductivity. The degree to which it can be polarized, either by the creation of new dipoles or by the co-orientation of permanently dipolar molecules, is a measure of its permittivity.

Ex vivo data show that electrical property values can differ by a factor of 5 to 10 between normal and malignant human breast tissues over the microwave frequency range [21, 22]. Malignant mammary tumors apparently have electrical properties which mimic those typically found in high-water-content tissues such as muscle, whereas normal breast has properties typical of low-water-content, fatty tissues. The increased blood volume associated with the neovascularization of the rapidly proliferating tumor periphery may be responsible for increased water content, a variable to which microwave illumination is particularly sensitive. In fact, one study has found that for normal and malignant human tissues of the same histological type, greater differences in electrical properties occur in mammary than in colon, kidney, liver, lung, and muscle [17].

In short, EM properties in the microwave band offer high intrinsic contrast for pathology, especially in the breast. Exploiting this contrast for imaging has been challenging because of the difficulties associated with inducing and measuring a response noninvasively that can be used to discriminate local variations in EM properties. However, our MIS effort has met a number of these challenges and is poised to complete the first critical evaluation of the potential of microwave breast imaging. A clinical imaging system has been realized that transceives broadband, high-fidelity propagating fields through a noncontacting antenna array translated axially under computer control; this system will deliver MIS exams to pendant breasts immersed in a fluid that promotes signal coupling.

2.4   Near Infrared Spectroscopic Imaging (NIS)

In NIS, a circular array of optodes (in this case, optical fibers transceiving infrared laser light) is placed in contact with the pendant breast. Each optode in turn is used to illuminate the interior of the breast, serving as a detector when nonactive. A two- or three-dimensional FE model of the breast's optical properties is iteratively optimized until simulated observations based on the model converge with observation.

Published data have long supported the notion that near infrared spectroscopy and imaging offer excellent contrast potential. Studies have shown 2:1 contrast between excised tumor and normal breast at certain near infrared wavelengths [23, 24]. Correlations with increase in blood vessel number and size (which is characteristic of neovascularization in the tumor periphery and may lead to a fourfold increase in blood volume) have been reported [25] and have been estimated to translate into 4:1 contrast in optical absorption coefficients [26] (see Sec. 3, "Correlation With Pathology").

In addition to the absorption contrast afforded by blood-concentration changes in tumorigenic regions of the breast, contrast specificity provided by light scattering resulting from calcifications involving matrix accumulation of insoluble phosphates, often associated with tumors, may also be exploitable for imaging purposes [27]. The detailed forms of microcalcifications would not be visible due to spatial resolution limits, but the aggregate optical signature of calcification clusters may be detectable. Another potential contrast mechanism is provided by the lipid content of the tissue, the spectral peaks of which occur at 750 nm and 940 nm; these peaks would presumably be reduced in breast cancers as compared to surrounding, normal, fattier tissue. It is furthermore notable that the optical properties imaged spectrally with NIS — absorption and scatter — can be used to deduce certain physiological variables, such as total hemoglobin concentration and oxygen saturation. These are being investigated as possible means to differentiate benign from malignant breast disease (see Ch. 10).

Our NIS initiative has been the first of our modality initiatives to regularly employ three-dimensional data acquisition and image reconstruction during clinical breast exams. Further, it has led the way in terms of analyzing its imaging data in both the normal and abnormal breast in relation to clinical factors and histological indicators in order to explore and explain the biological/physiological basis of image contrast. It has also pioneered the overall movement within our program toward image assessment by both quantitative methods (contrast-to-noise metrics) and qualitative methods (observer experiments) in order to characterize how nonlinear image reconstruction influences traditional contrast-detail and region-of-interest curves.

3   CORRELATION WITH PATHOLOGY

A distinguishing feature of these imaging modalities is that they recover actual tissue property distributions that provide functional information about the tissue being interrogated. A crucial aspect of this multi-modality project is the investigation of the relationship between the imaged properties and actual tissue pathology. Toward this end, the following section describes initial pathology studies that have been conducted in parallel with imaging modality development. A general overview of breast physiology is followed by a more in-depth discussion of morphologic criteria that may correlate with contrast mechanisms operative in alternative imaging modalities. The discussion is somewhat technical, so non-medical readers may wish to skip directly to Section 4, "Unifying the Four Modalities."

3.1   The Breast

The adult female breast is a large, modified sebaceous gland that consists mostly of fat, fibrous septa, and glandular structures. The weight range for a "normal," mature female breast is 30 grams to over 500 grams, depending on the woman's body habitus. The breast typically comprises 15 to 25 lobes that are divided into multiple lobules, each containing 10–100 terminal milk-secreting alveoli. Numerous tiny milk-transporting ductules combine to form a single lactiferous duct that exits each lobule. About 15 to 25 such ducts converge at the nipple. The composition of the breast varies from individual to individual and with age and other factors. Pregnancy, lactation, menstruation, and menopause all introduce characteristic changes in breast physiology. For example, in postmenopausal involution of the breast, the lobular and alveolar structures regress and the vascularity of the intervening connective tissue is reduced. Eventually only small, occasional islands of functional breast parenchyma remain, surrounded by dense, scarred connective tissue [28].

3.2   Breast Tissue Morphology

We have only a limited understanding of the biological and physiological bases of image contrast for malignancy and their relation to biological and molecular markers of cancer progression or regression that are predictive of therapeutic response and, ultimately, outcome. The interpretation and significance of variables imaged using alternative modalities will only be appreciated if the electromechanical properties being measured (e.g., electrical conductivity and permittivity, optical absorption and scattering, and mechanical elasticity and compressibility) are correlated with the biological characteristics of the tissue being imaged. Measures of tissue microvascularity such as mean vessel density and area may correlate with hemoglobin concentration and oxygen saturation, as indirectly measured by NIS. The ratio of functional breast parenchymal epithelium to surrounding dense connective tissue stroma (epithelium-to-stroma ratio, E:S) may correlate with tissue hardness, elasticity or compressibility as measured by MRE. Variable interfaces between tissue types are also likely to influence the electromagnetic properties associated with modalities such as EIS and MIS, which are sensitive to such morphologic attributes of the local cell population as volume fraction, membrane integrity, water content, and ionic concentrations. Unfortunately, biological correlates with tissue water content are difficult to evaluate since the tissue must be routinely processed (formalin-fixed, dehydrated, and paraffin-embedded) in order not to compromise the pathologist's ability to make a definitive tissue diagnosis.

A range of electromechanical and biological values for *normal* breast tissue must first be established to ensure a meaningful comparison to *diseased* breast tissue. To this end, we have completed a study employing a computer-aided program specifically developed to reproducibly assess microvasculature and tissue type interfaces in benign and malignant breast tissue.

The benign diagnostic categories comprised (1) breast tissue with normal histology, (2) fibrocystic disease, and (3) a common benign neoplasm (fibroadenoma). The malignant neoplasm category comprised invasive carcinomas. Fourteen patients who underwent breast-reduction surgery with sampling from both breasts provided tissue with normal breast histology. Twenty-one patients (16 of whom also underwent breast reduction surgery with sampling from both breasts, 5 with unilateral biopsies) provided tissue with fibrocystic disease of variable severity (mild, moderate, or severe). Nineteen patients provided tissue with a benign fibroadenoma from one breast, each lesion classified according to the degree of stromal hyalinization or scarring in the tumor. Seventeen patients provided tissue with an invasive, malignant carcinoma from one breast [29].

Mean vessel density (MVD, percentage of each unit area that consists of transected vessels), mean vessel area (MVA, average cross-sectional area of an individual vessel), and vessel orientation (correlated with shape of observed cross-section) were the morphologic criteria chosen to assess tissue microvascularity. The criteria chosen to evaluate tissue hardness, elasticity, and compressibility were the epithelium-to-stroma ratio (E:S), the degree of severity of fibrocystic disease, the degree of stromal hyalinization or scarring in the benign neoplasms (fibroadenomas), the infiltrative patterns of the malignant neoplasms (carcinomas), and the type of tissue interfacing with the neoplasms (fatty, fibrofatty, fibrous, fibrocystic changes).

Computerized image-processing techniques can be used to select regions of interest in tissue samples for analysis. First, hematoxylin and eosin are used to stain routinely processed (i.e., formalin-fixed, paraffin-embedded) tissue sections. The segmentation of specific regions of interest (vessels and epithelium) is facilitated if these regions are stained to distinguish them from the surrounding tissues. Outlining of vessels can then be achieved using a specific immunologic marker of the endothelial cells that line the vessels (i.e., a commercially available CD31 stain). The epithelial component of the tissue can be distinguished from the surrounding connective tissue stroma using a specific immunologic marker of epithelial cells (cytokeratin 5D3).

Using these immunohistochemical techniques, we analyzed more than 100 breast specimens for MVD, MVA, shape,* and E:S across the four diagnostic categories, namely (1) normal, (2) fibrocystic disease, (3) benign neoplasms (fibroadenomas), and (4) malignant neoplasms (invasive carcinomas). Representative micrographs illustrating tissue types, computer processing, and staining are given in Figures 1–4. Vessel analysis of the neoplasms was compared peripherally and centrally. Adjusted t-tests assessed the effects of fibroadenoma stromal hyalinization or scarring and fibrocystic disease severity. Measurement reproducibility for the three benign diagnostic groups was assessed using Spearman correlation coefficients.

	Normal	Fibro-cystic disease	Fibroadenoma $N = 19$		Cancer $N = 17$	
	$N = 28$	$N = 37$	Peripheral	Central	Peripheral	Central
Mean vessel area (MVA)*	125 (115–136)	122 (113–131)	182 (164–202)	177 (160–196)	139 (120–162)	136 (116–158)
E:S*	0.013 (0.009–0.018)	0.028 (0.021–0.037)	0.069 (0.055–0.087)		0.162 (0.127–0.206)	
Shape*	0.45 (0.43–0.46)	0.43 (0.42–0.44)	0.40 (0.38–0.41)	0.39 (0.38–0.41)	0.44 (0.42–0.45)	0.44 (0.42–0.45)
Microvessel density (MVD)*	0.27 (0.17–0.36)	0.42 (0.34–0.50)	0.49 (0.40–0.58)	0.40 (0.31–0.49)	0.77 (0.68–0.86)	0.76 (0.67–0.85)

* $p < .001$.

Table 1. Adjusted means with confidence intervals for the variables in normal breast, fibrocystic disease, fibroadenomas, and carcinomas. Values in bold are means. Ranges are in parentheses are 95% confidence intervals. E:S = epithelium-to-stroma ratio. Units of MVA are μ^2.

---

* Equivalent to vessel orientation. "Shape" is a unitless measure of a vessel's elliptical cross-section, calculated as the length of the ellipse's minor axis divided by the length of its major axis. For example, a vessel of circular cross section has a shape of 1; a vessel cut at such an angle that its cross-section is an ellipse twice as long as it is wide has a shape of .5.

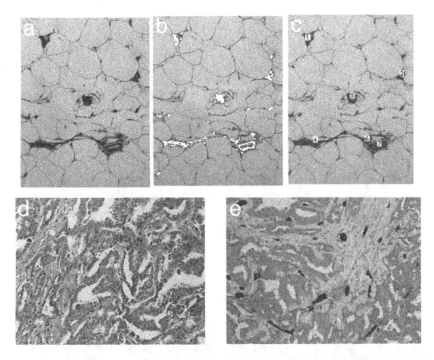

Figure 1. Immunostaining of normal breast tissue with the pan-endothelial marker CD31 highlights the endothelium-lined vessels per unit area (a). Using gray-value segmentation (b), the endothelial-lined vessels with positive immunostaining are automatically outlined and counted (c). Dedicated image-processing macros then provide the microvessel density (MVD), microvessel area (MVA), and total vessel count per unit area. As compared to a mean MVD of 0.27 (SD 0.095) for normal breast, the mean MVD for an infiltrating ductal carcinoma (d and e) is 0.77 (SD 0.09). Hematoxylin and eosin stain (d), CD31 immunostaining (e).

The adjusted means for the chosen morphologic variables in normal breast, fibrocystic disease, fibroadenomas, and carcinomas are given in Table 1. There is a significant difference between the value ranges for MVD, MVA, E:S, and shape when comparing the four diagnostic categories ($p < .001$). For the invasive carcinomas, the significances for E:S and MVD were higher ($p < .001$) as compared to fibroadenomas, but that for MVA was smaller. When comparing the fibroadenomas and carcinomas centrally versus peripherally, there was no significant difference between the four measured variables.

Correlation coefficients for method reproducibility were high across the diagnostic categories: E:S, 0.90–0.94; MVD, 0.92–0.96; MVA, 0.61–0.78; vessel shape, 0.61–0.90. There was right-versus-left (breast) predictability for MVD only in normal breast. In fibrocystic disease, three variables (E:S,

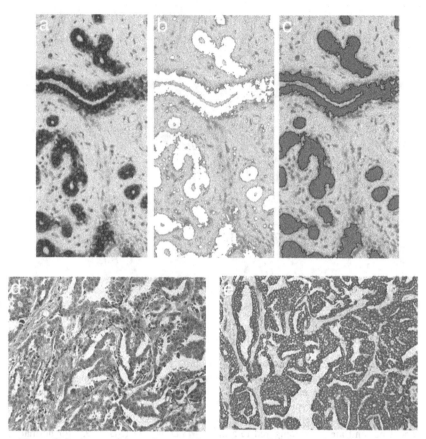

Figure 2. Immunostaining of normal breast tissue with the cytokeratin 5D3 high-lights the epithelial components (a). Using gray-value segmentation (b), the areas of epithelium with positive immunostaining are outlined (c) and measured as a ratio of the surrounding, unstained stroma to derive the epithelium-to-stroma ratio (E:S). As compared to a mean E:S of 0.013 (SD 0.0045) for normal breast, the mean E:S for an infiltrating ductal carcinoma (d, e) is 0.162 (SD 0.0395). Hematoxylin and eosin stain (d), cytokeratin immunostaining (e).

MVA, and vessel shape) showed right-versus-left predictability, most significantly for E:S ($p < .001$).

Of the 37 cases of fibrocystic disease, 7 samples (each with right and left specimens) were classified with mild fibrocystic changes (1+), 9 samples (each with right and left specimens) with moderate changes (2+), and the remaining 5 samples (unilateral specimens) with severe changes (3+). The trend of an increasing E:S with increased severity of fibrocystic disease ($p < .001$) reflects the associated proliferation of epithelium. These findings may influence the ability to detect a breast cancer given a background of severe fibrocystic changes as compared to fat. The degree of fibrocystic disease

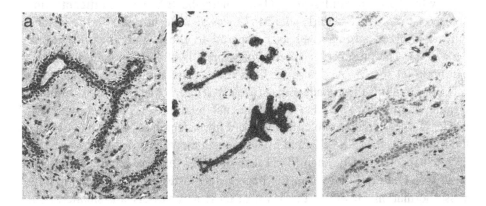

Figure 3. For this benign fibroadenoma with hyalinized stroma, shown with hematoxylin and eosin stain (a), 1.4 cm in diameter and interfacing with fat, computer-assisted image processing of cytokeratin 5D3 immunostaining (b) gave an E:S of 0.05. Analysis of immunostaining with the pan-endothelial marker CD31 (c) gave an MVD of 0.45 and an MVA of 175 μ^2.

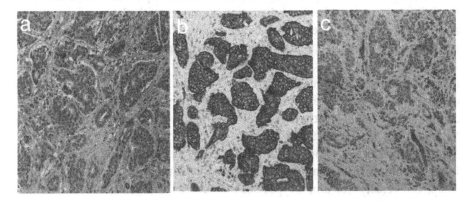

Figure 4. For this infiltrating ductal carcinoma of intermediate grade, 0.8 cm diameter, and interfacing with fat, shown in (a) with hematoxylin and eosin stain, computer-assisted image processing of cytokeratin 5D3 immunostaining (b) gave an E:S of 0.119. Analysis of pan-endothelial marker CD31 immunostaining (c) gave an MVD of 0.68 and an MVA of 155 μ^2.

did not affect the MVD but the MVA decreased as the severity of fibrocystic disease increased ($p = .038$).

Of the 19 fibroadenomas measured in our study, 6 were classified with predominantly loose, myxoid stroma (1+), 5 with predominantly hyalinized (scarred) stroma (3+), and 8 with a mixture of both stroma types (2+). In the fibroadenomas with more stromal hyalinization (3+), the proportional amounts of associated epithelium were less as compared to the fibroadenomas with loose, myxoid stroma (1+), where the E:S was significantly increased ($p < .001$). Similarly, the MVD was significantly less in the lesions with hyalinized stroma (3+) as compared to those with myxoid stroma ($p < .001$). The presence or absence of stromal hyalinization did not significantly affect the MVA. These findings may be important in distinguishing sclerotic, hyalinized fibroadenomas (usually seen in older patients) from malignant neoplasms. We also postulate that hyalinized fibroadenomas are harder and less compressible than myxoid fibroadenomas, which may impact the findings of the EIS, MIS, and MRE imaging modalities.

As expected, the E:S and MVD seen in the 17 invasive breast carcinomas were significantly higher than the benign diagnostic groups, reflecting new vessel formation. However, the MVA of these new vessels was smaller, both peripherally and centrally, in the malignant neoplasms than in the benign neoplasms. Of the 17 carcinomas measured in the current study, 14 were usual infiltrating ductal carcinomas, 2 were lobular carcinomas, and one was a colloid or mucinous carcinoma (a variant of a ductal carcinoma with a high mucin component). We postulate that the infiltrative pattern of a tumor and its ability to cause architectural distortion correlates with changes seen in imaging modalities. The sclerotic, spiculated mass of a typical ductal carcinoma would most likely cause greater compression changes than the single-cell, insidious growth pattern of a lobular carcinoma or the soft, well-circumscribed mass of a colloid/mucinous carcinoma (which causes only minimal distortion of the surrounding tissue). We also postulate that a typical invasive ductal carcinoma arising in a fatty breast will exhibit a more sharply contrasting attenuation signal at the tumor/fat interface than the same tumor arising in dense, fibrous breast stroma. In the latter case, the attenuation gradient (i.e., in transitioning from tumor to collagen to surrounding fat) would be less steep. Conversely, for tumor types such as tubular or lobular, which infiltrate as subtle tubules or single cells respectively, it is likely that signal attenuation would be more diffuse and the proportions of epithelium (tumor and normal) to connective tissue stroma and to fat less well-defined.

The results for shape (vessel orientation), where ranges of 0–1 correlate with perfectly longitudinal and perfectly transverse vessel sectioning respectively, suggest near-random alignment of the vascular spaces in benign and malignant breast tissue. Overall, vessel shape values were significantly lower in the fibroadenomas than the other diagnostic categories, representing a trend towards a more longitudinal arrangement.

This study has a number of limitations. Tissue fixation and dehydration prevent the evaluation of water content and other criteria; small tissue samples may not be representative of larger volumes; the areas evaluated in each sample are not randomly selected by a computer-driven slide stage; method reproducibility for multiple observers has not been evaluated; and the malignant tumors used for comparison with the benign breast tissue were all invasive carcinomas. Nevertheless, this study establishes a reproducible computer-assisted technique to assess morphologic criteria in benign and malignant breast tissue that may correlate with properties detected by alternative breast imaging techniques. It also provides a baseline of expected values for normal and abnormal breast tissue against which results from study subjects can be compared. In this regard, pathological findings in 39 study subjects with biopsied screening abnormalities have been evaluated. The morphometric measurements from the study subjects fall within the ranges established in Table 1. The measures from the initial core biopsies are occasionally lower than either the established normal ranges or the subsequent excisional biopsies, due to limited sampling in the cores. (Excisional biopsy specimens were used to establish the data in Table 1.)

In an additional set of analyses, we compared pathology measures to electromechanical properties as determined by alternative imaging modalities. Table 2 reports Spearman correlations between pathology and imaged properties for regions of interest from exams with abnormal conventional findings. These correlation coefficients suggest possible relationships between property measures and specific pathological properties of the related biopsy material. In particular, we note a fairly high correlation between vessel density and the NIS-derived value for Hb_T (total hemoglobin). The relationship between pathological vessel density and percent blood determined from imaged NIS parameters is particularly clear (Figure 5).

Cross-modality correlations have also been investigated (Table 3). Interestingly, most cross-modality property correlations are modest, suggesting that each method is sensitive to different tissue characteristics in the region of interest. Note, however, that water percentage from the NIS data is strongly correlated with MIS permittivity. This is intuitively satisfying, since MIS permittivity is known to be sensitive to water content, and confirms that the two methods are recovering important information about tissue composition. The amount of localized property enhancement associated with cancer in the various modalities is discussed further in Chapter 11.

Pathology		NIS					MIS		EIS	
		Hb_T (μM)	S_1O_2 (%)	Water (%)	Scatter power	Scatter amp.	ε_r	σ	ε_r	σ
MVA	r_s	0.224	-0.557	-0.273	0.294	0.361	0.179	0.028	0.124	0.082
	p	0.48	0.060	0.42	0.35	0.25	0.56	0.93	0.60	0.73
E:S	r_s	0.467	0.258	0.713	0.214	0.198	0.134	-0.371	-0.249	-0.143
	p	0.11	0.39	0.009	0.48	0.52	0.65	0.19	0.28	0.54
Shape	r_s	0.490	-0.413	-0.355	0.231	0.315	-0.132	-0.484	0.559	-0.129
	p	0.11	0.18	0.28	0.47	0.32	0.67	0.094	0.010	0.59
MVD	r_s	0.713	-0.308	-0.036	0.517	0.524	-0.099	-0.615	0.147	-0.293
	p	0.009	0.33	0.092	0.085	0.080	0.75	0.025	0.54	0.21

Table 2. Spearman correlations (r_s) between pathology measures and imaged properties for regions of interest from exams with abnormal conventional findings. The p-value for each correlation is also given. MVA = microvessel area (units of μ^2); E:S = epithelium-to-stroma ratio; MVD = microvessel density; Hb_T = total hemoglobin; S_1O_2 = tissue hemoglobin oxygen saturation. Note $p < .009$ for correlation of MVD to NIS-derived value for Hb_T.

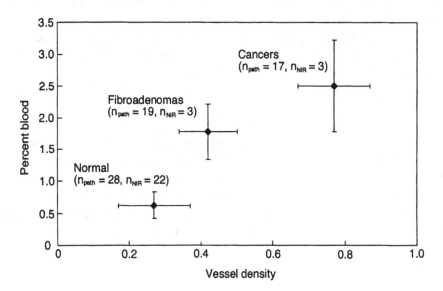

Figure 5. Relationship between pathological vessel density (MVD, expressed as a number between 0 and 1 rather than as a percentage) and percent blood, as determined from imaged NIS parameters. Error bars show the standard deviations in both dimensions.

			NIS					EIS	
			Hb_T (μM)	S_tO_2 (%)	Water (%)	Scatter power	Scatter amp.	ε_r	σ
MIS	ε_r	r_P	0.43	0.25	0.80	0.069	0.065	0.18	0.15
		p	0.16	0.43	0.003	0.83	0.84	0.56	0.63
	σ	r_P	-0.29	-0.24	0.37	-0.19	-0.19	-0.20	0.41
		p	0.36	0.45	0.26	0.56	0.56	0.51	0.17
EIS	ε_r	r_P	0.067	-0.015	-0.27	0.20	0.19	-	-
		p	0.84	0.96	0.43	0.52	0.55	-	-
	σ	r_P	-0.020	-0.27	-0.085	-0.39	-0.36	-	-
		p	0.95	0.40	0.80	0.21	0.25	-	-

Table 3. Pearson correlation coefficients (r_P) and associated p-values for modality-specific properties. Hb_T = total hemoglobin; S_tO_2 = tissue hemoglobin oxygen saturation.

An additional remark concerning the MVD measure is called for. We originally selected mean MVD as a morphometric measure following work by Weidner et al. [30], who showed that increased MVD (>100 per $200\times$ field) in early-stage invasive node-negative breast carcinoma was an independent prognostic indicator for reduced overall survival and recurrence-free survival. However, as the review article by Hlatky et al. eloquently reminds us [31], microvessel density does not reflect the angiogenic activity or angiogenic dependence of a tumor. It is really a measure of "intercapillary distance" (i.e., the number of vessels per unit area), which is determined by the net balance between the effects of stimulatory and inhibitory angiogenic factors on vessel growth as well as by non-angiogenic factors such as oxygen- and nutrient-consumption rates. In particular, the number of tumor cells that can be supported by a vessel depends on the metabolic needs of those cells; the higher the rate of oxygen and nutrient consumption, the smaller the number of tumor cells that can squeeze between capillaries without becoming necrotic. This, in turn, influences the vascular density (intercapillary distance). MVD therefore varies markedly with tumor type. Some tumors (e.g., those of the lung, colon, and kidney), despite considerable angiogenic activity, exhibit *lower* microvessel densities than surrounding normal tissues. Therefore, despite its importance as a prognostic indicator in untreated tumors, a low intratumoral MVD is not a sufficient criterium to exclude a patient from treatment with angiogenesis inhibitors.

The pan-endothelial cell immunomarker CD31, which we used to measure MVD, labels both the activated endothelial cells lining newly formed vessels and the endothelial cells lining vessels established since embryogenesis. MVD evaluated using CD31 needs to be validated against MVD evaluated using immunomarkers specific for activated endothelial cells only, such as the endothelial membrane glycoprotein endoglin (CD105) and the integral membrane metalloprotease CD13. MVD also needs to be correlated with other markers of angiogenic activity, including angiogenic peptides such as vascular endothelial growth factor (VEGF) and basic fibroblast growth factor (bFGF); matrix-degrading proteolytic enzymes such as urokinase-type plasminogen (uPA) and plasminogen activator inhibitor I (PAI-1); and plasminogen-activated cytokines such as transforming growth factor beta (TGF-beta).

4   UNIFYING THE FOUR MODALITIES

The importance of developing alternative breast cancer imaging modalities is that they may access new mechanisms of physiological contrast. Further, there may be synergistic effects when the four approaches discussed in this text are used as complements to each other rather than in isolation. This multimodality approach is an important theme, as it is unlikely that any single breast-imaging method will be superior across the whole spectrum of women receiving clinical breast care.

With this approach in mind, the clinical introduction of these alternative modalities is being coordinated by our clinical research team at the Dartmouth-Hitchcock Medical Center. The clinical team supplies the infrastructure for efficient subject recruitment and for the generation of a common database of clinical experiences, image analyses, case studies, and outcomes. This enables us to compare alternative and conventional imaging modalities in a common set of clinical circumstances and to compare the information obtained from using multiple modalities to that gained from each modality alone.

In addition to assessing whether there is a synergistic diagnostic effect when combining all four approaches, the projects are working to pool their computational resources where possible. This not only minimizes costly overlap but also facilitates cross-fertilization of new methods that may benefit all modalities. As mentioned earlier, each modality utilizes an iterative technique for recovering the property images. All apply FE modeling to achieve efficient calculation of the governing partial differential equations and complex reconstruction techniques. These techniques involve advanced numerical algorithmic concepts, making them critically dependant on the robust software implementation and access to state-of-the-art computing environment that are provided by our computational team.

While this framework is clearly useful, development within each individual project retains important independent aspects, particularly in relation to the unique physical requirements of each. In this book, this balance of coordination and individuality is reflected in the computational overview in Chapter 2 and the treatises on the theory and numerical implementation specific to each modality (Chapters 3, 5, 7, and 9).

Figure 6 illustrates the development interactions of the four modalities and the supporting clinical and computational teams (or "cores"). The circular path connecting the individual modality projects represents the flow of information that may originate in any one project and influence one or more of the others. Such influence is possible because, while each modality project is responsible for its own technological advancement, preclinical testing/evaluation, and clinical image analysis, all four projects pursue quantitative breast tissue property mapping that consists of the same three essential elements: (1) a controlled stimulus applied to the breast over a three-dimensional volume encompassing the region of interest; (2) fast, accurate

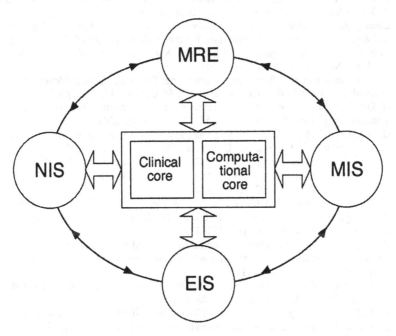

Figure 6. Relation of the four modalities to the clinical and computational cores.

measurement of breast response to the applied stimulus over the corresponding tissue volume; and (3) image formation from the response based on breast property parameter estimations achieved through mathematical modeling techniques. As a result, interactions and collaborations between project components exist in areas of hardware/software data generation, acquisition, calibration, and validation along with image reconstruction and analysis.

5   A GLANCE AHEAD

The next chapter expounds the significant computational ground held in common by all four modalities. The remainder of the book will take a closer look at the mathematics, hardware, and results of each of the four modalities. A pair of chapters is devoted to each modality, one to explore computational and theoretical issues and another to describe devices and results.

REFERENCES

[1]   L. A. G. Rise et al., *SEER Cancer Statistics Review 1973–1994.* NIH Publication No. 97-2789 (Bethesda, MD: National Cancer Institute, 1994).

[2]   Committee on Technologies for the Early Detection of Breast Cancer, *Mammography and Beyond: Developing Technologies for the Early Detection of Breast Cancer*, S. J. Nass, I. C. Henderson, and J. C. Lashof, eds., National Cancer Policy Board (Washington, D.C.: National Academy Press, 2001).

[3]   L. L. Humphrey et al., "Breast cancer screening: Summary of the evidence for the U.S. Preventive Services Task Force." *Ann. Intern . Med.*, Vol. 137, 2002, pp. 347–360.

[4]   O. Olsen and P. C. Gøtzsche, "Cochrane review of screening for breast cancer with mammography" (letter). *Lancet*, Vol. 358, 2001, pp. 1340–1342.

[5]   O. Olsen and P. C. Gøtzsche, "Systematic review of screening for breast cancer with mammography." The Nordic Cochrane Center, Denmark, 2001, available at http://image.thelancet.com/lancet/extra/fullreport/pdf (accessed Jan. 29, 2004).

[6]   S. W. Fletcher et al., "Report of the International Workshop on Screening for Breast Cancer." *JNCI*, Vol. 85, 1993, 1644–1656.

[7]   US Preventive Service Task Force, *Ann. Intern. Med.*, Vol. 137, 2002, pp. 344–346.

[8]   P. T. Huynh, A. M. Jarolimek, and S. Daye, "The false-negative mammogram." *Radiographics*, Vol. 18, No. 5, 1998, pp. 1137–1154.

[9]   P. A. Carney et al., "Individual and combined effects of age, breast density and hormone replacement therapy use on the accuracy of screening mammography." *Ann. Intern. Med.*, Vol. 138, 2003, pp. 168–175.

[10]   N. F. Boyd et al., "Quantitative classification of mammographic densities and breast cancer risk," *JNCI*, Vol. 87, 1995, pp. 670–675.

[11]   E. A. Sickles, "Nonpalpable, circumscribed, noncalcified, solid breast masses: Likelihood of malignancy based on lesion size and age of patient." *Radiology*, Vol. 192, 1994, pp. 439–442.

[12] C. Byrne et al., "Survival advantage differences by age. Evaluation of the extended follow-up of the Breast Cancer Detection Demonstration Project." *Cancer: Diagnosis, Treatment, Research*, July 1994 (1 Suppl), pp. 301–310.

[13] F. Lee Jr. et al., "Sonoelasticity imaging: Results in *in vitro* tissue specimens." *Radiology*, Vol. 181(1), 1991, pp. 237–239.

[14] M. A. Hadley et al., "Sonoelasticity imaging of prostate cancer." *RSNA Abstracts*, 1993.

[15] D. J. Rubens et al., "Sonoelasticity imaging of prostate cancer: *In vitro* results." *Radiology*, Vol. 195(2), 1995, pp. 379–385.

[16] J. Cuzick et al., "Electropotential measurements as a new diagnostic modality for breast cancer." *Lancet*, Vol. 352, 1998, pp. 359–363.

[17] T. Morimoto et al., "Measurement of the electrical bioimpedance of breast tumors." *Eur. Surg. Res.*, Vol. 22, 1990, pp. 86–92.

[18] T. Morimoto et al., "A study of the electrical bioimpedance of tumors." *J. Invest. Surg.*, Vol. 6, 1993, pp. 25–32.

[19] J. Jossinet, "Variability of impedivity in normal and pathological breast tissue." *Med. & Biol. Eng. & Comput.*, Vol. 34, 1996, pp. 346–350.

[20] A. J. Surowiec et al., "Dielectric properties of breast carcinoma and the surrounding tissues." *IEEE Trans. Biomed. Eng.*, Vol. 35, 1988, pp. 257–263.

[21] W. T. Joines et al., "The measured electrical properties of normal and malignant human tissues from 50 to 90 MHz." *Med. Phys.*, Vol. 21, 1994, pp. 547–550.

[22] S. S. Chaudhary et al., "Dielectric properties of normal and malignant human breast tissues at radiowave and microwave frequencies." *Indian J. Biochem. Biophys.*, Vol. 21, 1984, pp. 76–79.

[23] V. G. Peters et al., "Optical properties of normal and diseased human breast tissue in the visible and near infrared." *Phys. Med. Biol.*, Vol. 35, 1990, pp. 1317–1334.

[24] H. Key, "Optical attenuation characteristics of breast tissues at visible and near-infrared wavelengths." *Phys. Med. Biol.*, Vol. 36, 1991, pp. 579–590.

[25] A. E. Profio, G. A. Navarro, and O. W. Sartorius, "Scientific basis of breast diaphanography." *Med. Phys.*, Vol. 16, 1989, pp. 60–65.

[26] B. W. Pogue et al., "Initial assessment of a simple system for frequency-domain diffuse optical tomography." *Phys. Med. Biol.*, Vol. 40, 1995, pp. 1709–1729.

[27] B. Chance et al., "On the medical uses of photon migration in tissues," in *Integration of Medical Optical Imaging and Spectroscopy and Magnetic Resonance Imaging Symposium Abstracts*, Dec. 2, Philadelphia, PA, 1994.

[28] S. S. Sternberg, ed., *Histology for Pathologists*, 2nd Ed., Ch. 4 (Philadelphia: Lippencott Raven Publishers, 1997). [This note applies to the whole foregoing paragraph.]

[29] W. Wells et al., "Analysis of the microvasculature and tissue type ratios in normal vs. benign and malignant breast tissue." *Journal of Analytical and Quantitative Cytology and Histology*, Vol. 26, 2004, pp. 166-174.

[30] N. Weidner et al., "Tumor angiogenesis: A new significant and independent prognostic indicator in early-stage breast carcinoma." *JNCI*, Vol. 84(24), 1992, 1875-1887.

[31] L. Hlatlky, P. Hahnfeldt, and J. Folkman, "Clinical application of antiangiogenic therapy: Microvessel density, what it does and doesn't tell us." *JNCI*, Vol. 94(12), 2002, 883-893.

Chapter 2

COMPUTATIONAL FRAMEWORK

Paul M. Meaney, Ph.D. and Keith Paulsen, Ph.D.

1   INTRODUCTION

All of the imaging modalities discussed in this book require unique numerical algorithms and data acquisition hardware. However, they also share a good deal of algorithmic common ground. The Dartmouth Breast Imaging Group has therefore articulated a shared numerical-analysis framework for these modalities. This framework facilitates communication between teams working on different modalities while being flexible enough to allow for needful variations, especially as dictated by the data-acquisition requirements of each modality.

In all four modalities, imaging requires the solution of an inverse problem. That is, measurements are made of some physical process (e.g., microwaves, infrared light, or mechanical vibrations) that interacts with the tissue, and from these external recordings the two- or three-dimensional distribution of physical properties of the tissue (dielectric properties, optical absorption coefficient, elasticity) is estimated using numerical algorithms.

The imaging strategies used by three of the modalities—electrical impedance spectroscopy (EIS), microwave imaging spectroscopy (MIS), and near-infrared spectroscopic imaging (NIS)—resemble those of x-ray computed tomography (CT). That is, they collect data with an array of detectors positioned around a central target while illuminating the target successively from all directions. The fourth modality, magnetic resonance elastography (MRE), is distinctly nontomographic in that it excites the whole tissue volume using a piezoelectric-based mechanical vibration system and collects displacement information at each voxel within the target using magnetic resonance imaging techniques.

Because x-rays propagate in nearly straight lines through tissue, in CT an attenuation coefficient can be assigned directly to each pixel. The inverse solution for these attenuation coefficients requires only linear matrix operations. For the imaging modalities treated in this book, however, the inverse problem is nonlinear, because the physical interactions do not occur along straight lines but rather are distributed essentially throughout the imaging field-of-view. As a result, the measured response is not a linear function of tissue properties and iterative numerical methods are required to solve the inversion problem.

We have chosen to apply a well-known iterative technique, the Gauss-Newton method, to the solution of this suite of nonlinear inverse problems [1]. We estimate the spatial distribution of the tissue's physical properties; calculate the response that *would* be observed, given this distribution (i.e., solve the "forward problem"); compare these calculated observations to the actual data; and update the estimated property distribution accordingly. This process is iterated until the real and calculated observations converge, whereupon the estimated distribution is taken as the desired image.

2   FORWARD PROBLEM

2.1   Field Equations

Our finite-element approach requires that the measurable physical phenomenon of interest (e.g., electromagnetic waves) must be governed by a partial differential equation. Listed below are the model equations for the four modalities, along with the tissue properties associated with the measurable responses.

1. *Helmholtz wave equation* (MIS). For sinusoidal electromagnetic waves in source-free regions, Maxwell's equations reduce to the homogeneous Helmholtz wave equations [2]. In particular, the electric-field component **E** of a sinusoidal electromagnetic wave obeys

$$\nabla^2 \mathbf{E} + k^2 \mathbf{E} = 0 \qquad (2.1)$$

Here $k^2 = \omega^2 \mu \varepsilon + j \omega \mu \sigma$, where k is the wave number, ω is radian frequency, $j = \sqrt{-1}$, and the medium is characterized by magnetic permeability μ, electrical permittivity ε, and conductivity σ. In media with nonuniform electrical properties (e.g., tissue), k^2 varies locally. Its spatial variation throughout the breast is the quantity we are interested in imaging in MIS.

2. *Diffusion equation* (NIS). The diffusion equation for an absorptive, scattering, linearly anisotropic optical medium is

$$-\nabla \cdot D\nabla\Phi + \left(\mu_a + j\frac{\omega}{c_m} \right)\Phi = q_0 \qquad (2.2)$$

where Φ is the photon fluence, c_m is the speed of light in the medium, q_0 is the intensity of an isotropic light source, and D is the diffusion coefficient, which is a function of the absorption and reduced scattering coefficients μ_a and μ_s', i.e., $D = 1/[3(\mu_a + \mu_s')]$. The diffusion coefficient is the locally-varying physical quantity of interest in this modality.

3. *Laplace's equation* (EIS). In any charge-free region in a dielectric medium, the voltage (potential) at every point is governed by Laplace's equation:

$$\nabla \cdot (\sigma + j\omega\varepsilon)\nabla\Psi = 0 \qquad (2.3)$$

Here, Ψ is the voltage and the medium has electrical permittivity ε and conductivity σ. Laplace's equation is an appropriate relationship for EIS because the EIS system operates at frequencies several orders of magnitude below those used by the MIS system (a realm where the Helmholtz equation applies). As in MIS, the electrical properties of the tissue (ε and σ) are the physical quantities of interest.

4. *Navier's equation* (MRE). The governing differential relationship for the MRE modality is Navier's equation, which is in essence a multidimensional generalization of Hooke's Law of linear elasticity. Navier's equation describes the displacement field inside an elastic body subject throughout to stress and strain as follows:

$$\nabla \cdot \mu\nabla\mathbf{u} + \nabla(\lambda + \mu)\nabla \cdot \mathbf{u} = \rho\frac{\partial^2\mathbf{u}}{\partial t^2} \qquad (2.4)$$

Here, the three-dimensional vector $\mathbf{u}$ represents displacement within the medium, μ and λ are the material stiffness moduli known as Lamé's constants (presumed here to vary throughout the medium as scalar fields), and ρ is the density. The properties of interest are the moduli μ and λ (and possibly ρ).

For all modalities we have focused on the frequency-domain version of the problem; that is, we have assumed a periodic time variation of the form $e^{-i\omega t}$ for all nonconstant quantities and have solved the resulting steady-state system. An equally valid time-domain solution could be obtained on identical FE meshes by modeling the evolution of the system through time, but we have chosen the frequency-domain approach for the three tomographic modalities (MIS, NIS, EIS) because of limitations imposed by hardware calibration procedures and the advantages of exploiting the frequency-dispersion characteristics of the propagating media.*

For MRE, likewise, data are acquired at only a single mechanical-excitation frequency. Acquiring data at multiple mechanical excitation frequencies is possible but would be time-consuming using current methods.

2.2   Numerical Solution Framework

There are a number of numerical approaches for computing the electromagnetic fields or mechanical displacements throughout an inhomogeneous medium. These include finite elements, finite differences, method of moments, finite-difference time domain, and others [3–6]. Each has merits, but the finite element (FE) method is particularly useful for our purposes.

The FE method approximates a continuous medium as a mesh of polygonal or polyhedral elements with shared vertices (the nodes of the mesh). These elements are usually triangular (in 2D problems) or tetrahedral (in 3D problems). A basis function is centered on each node, and the physical phenomenon of interest is modeled at every point in the region of interest as a weighted sum of these basis functions. For an N-node mesh, this entails the solution of a matrix equation of the form $[A]\{\Phi\} = \{b\}$, where $[A]$ is $N \times N$; however, because the basis function associated with each node is nonzero only over those finite elements which contain that node, $[A]$ is sparse (populated with zeroes except near the diagonal) and therefore amenable to iterative and/or banded-matrix solutions. This enables important efficiencies in storage and computation [7]. Furthermore, the nodes of an FE mesh can be placed arbitrarily, allowing accurate modeling of irregular ob-

---

* Time-domain signals could be synthetically derived from frequency data by fast Fourier transform if it could be collected at a sufficiently large number of fixed frequencies, but this would dramatically increase hardware complexity and data-acquisition time. Conversely, the full-spectrum frequency response could be obtained from time-domain data.

ject contours and increased node density in areas where the fields to be modeled vary rapidly [4].

In the two-dimensional case (readily generalizable to three dimensions), we consider the physical phenomenon of interest (i.e., waves propagating through the image region) as a scalar field, $\Phi(x, y)$ (readily generalizable to a vector field). $\Phi(x, y)$ is defined over an area covered by a mesh of finite elements (Figure 1).

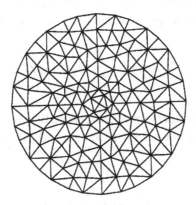

Figure 1. A two-dimensional finite-element mesh composed of several hundred triangular elements. In this particular mesh, each node (element vertex) is shared by as many as eight or as few as two elements.

Let $F[\Phi(x, y)] = 0$ be the differential equation (e.g., Laplace's) for which $\Phi(x, y)$ is the exact solution and for which some $\Phi_N(x, y)$, to be determined, is an *approximate* solution over an FE mesh having N nodes. $\Phi_N(x, y)$ is defined as the sum of N "basis functions," $\phi_i(x, y)$, that are weighted by N constants, Φ_i:

$$\Phi_N(x, y) = \sum_{i=1}^{N} \Phi_i\, \phi_i(x, y) \qquad (2.5)$$

The $\phi_i(x, y)$ are known and the N coefficients Φ_i are unknown.

In general, $F[\Phi_N(x, y)] = R$, the nonzero "residual" or error that results from substituting $\Phi_N(x, y)$ for the exact solution $\Phi(x, y)$. To minimize R, that is, to find the best possible $\Phi_N(x, y)$, we use the *weighted residual* method (described in many textbooks on finite element methods, e.g., [4]). In this approach, R is multiplied by a chosen weighting function $w_j(x, y)$, the product $w_j(x, y)R$ is integrated over the domain of the entire FE mesh, Ω, and the result is set equal to zero:

$$\int_{\Omega} w_j(x,y) R \, dx \, dy = 0 \qquad (2.6)$$

Substituting N different weighting functions $w_j(x,y)$ into (2.6) produces N equations in the N unknowns Φ_i.

Several simplifications can be made. First, each Lagrangian basis function $\phi_i(x,y)$ can be chosen to be nonzero only over those mesh elements of which the i th node is a vertex. Within each triangular finite element, therefore, only three $\phi_i(x,y)$ are nonzero and (2.5) simplifies to

$$\Phi_N(x,y) = \sum_{n=1}^{3} \Phi_n \phi_n(x,y) \qquad (2.7)$$

where n is a local index denoting the three vertices of the element, $\phi_n(x,y)$ is the basis function centered on node n, and Φ_n is the coefficient for $\phi_n(x,y)$ (see Figure 2).

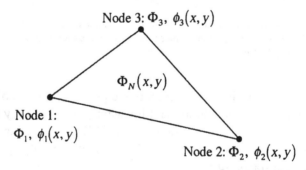

Figure 2. A triangular finite element. A coefficient Φ_n and linear basis function $\phi_n(x,y)$ are associated with each node. Each $\phi_n(x,y)$ is nonzero over this element and over all other elements of which its node is a vertex.

Second, in our implementation each basis function ϕ_i is linear, decreasing from 1 at the i th node to 0 along the opposite edge of each element sharing that node. The basis function ϕ_i at any node i that is surrounded entirely by mesh elements (i.e., any node that is not an edge node) can thus be visualized as an irregular pyramid with its peak over node i and its faces sloping down to the distal edges of all the elements sharing the node (Figure 3).

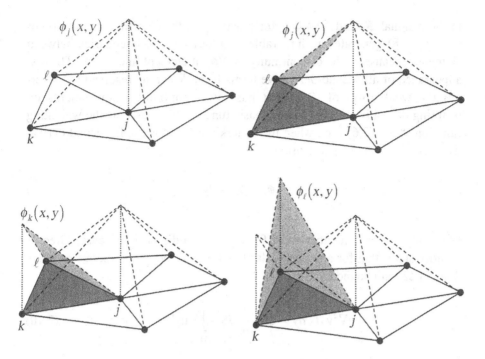

Figure 3. Relationship of piecewise-linear basis functions to triangular FE mesh elements. *Top left:* $\phi_j(x,y)$, the piecewise-linear basis function that is centered at node j, is shown over its whole domain (in this case, five elements). Its peak value is 1. *Top right:* The portion of $\phi_j(x,y)$ that overlaps element $jk\ell$ (dark gray). *Bottom left:* The portion of $\phi_k(x,y)$ that overlaps element $jk\ell$. *Bottom right:* The portion of $\phi_\ell(x,y)$ that overlaps element $jk\ell$. All other basis functions are zero over this element.

Third, the N basis functions ϕ_i used to form $\Phi_N(x,y)$ in (2.5) are employed as the N weighting functions w_i. When the weighting functions are equal to the basis functions, the resulting weighted-residuals method is termed the *Galerkin method.*

The presence of a Laplacian term (i.e., a second-order derivative) in the partial differential equation for each modality presents difficulties, since the basis functions are linear. That is, wherever a Laplacian term appears in the governing equation, it generates

$$\nabla^2 \Phi_N = \nabla^2 \left(\sum_{i=1}^{N} \Phi_i \phi_i \right) = \sum_{i=1}^{N} \Phi_i \nabla^2 \phi_i \tag{2.8}$$

in the residual R, and $\nabla^2 \phi_i = 0$ for linear ϕ_i on the element interior. (Technically, (2.8) generates an integrable singularity at the boundaries between elements because of the discontinuity in $\nabla \phi_i$ at element interfaces.) The disappearance of all second-derivative terms from R can be resolved by generating a weak form of (2.6) that has lower continuity requirements on resulting derivative terms. When a basis function ϕ_j is used as the weighting function w_j in (2.6) (i.e., when the Galerkin method is used), second derivatives like those in (2.8) give rise to

$$\int_\Omega \phi_j \nabla^2 \phi_i \, dx \, dy \tag{2.9}$$

We apply Green's identity to (2.9). In the two-dimensional case, Green's identity states that for any two scalar functions u and v continuous on some domain Ω with boundary C,

$$\int_\Omega u \nabla^2 v \, dx \, dy = \oint_C u \frac{\partial v}{\partial n} dS - \int_\Omega \nabla u \cdot \nabla v \, dx \, dy \tag{2.10}$$

where dS is a differential segment of C and $\partial v / \partial n = \nabla \phi_i \cdot \hat{\mathbf{n}}$ (i.e., the normal derivative) [4]. This yields

$$\langle \phi_j \nabla^2 \phi_i \rangle = \oint_C \frac{\partial \phi_i}{\partial n} \phi_j \, dS - \langle \nabla \phi_i \cdot \nabla \phi_j \rangle \tag{2.11}$$

where $\langle \cdot \rangle$ designates integration over the problem domain Ω. (In the three-dimensional case, $\langle \cdot \rangle$ designates volume integration and the contour integral becomes a surface integral.) Equation (2.11) contains derivatives of at most first order in both integral terms, sidestepping the problem of vanishing (singular) second-order derivatives. Another advantage of (2.11) is the appearance of the boundary integral, which is represented in terms of the natural boundary conditions expressed as the flux of the field through the enclosing surface.

When forcing and boundary conditions are taken into account, the resulting set of N weighted integral equations can be written in matrix form as

$$[A]\{\Phi\} = \{b\} \tag{2.12}$$

Matrix [A] is $N \times N$ and contains terms dependent on the governing equation. The vector of basis-function coefficients, $\{\Phi\} = \{\Phi_1, \Phi_2, \ldots \Phi_N\}$, is the quantity to be computed. The entries in $\{b\}$, which account for forcing functions (i.e., external inputs to the system) and boundary conditions, arise during evaluation of the contour integral in (2.11). Matrix [A] is sparse due to the localized nature of the basis functions, lending itself to efficient matrix-factorization routines [8] and/or iterative solvers.

Boundary conditions vary among modalities. For instance, the NIS and EIS approaches utilize mixed boundary conditions with

$$\Phi = A + B \frac{\partial \Phi}{\partial \mathbf{n}} \qquad (2.13)$$

Here, A and B are known constants and $\mathbf{n}$ is the unit normal vector oriented outward at the boundary [9]. The MRE approach applies either a Dirichlet or Neumann boundary conditions, depending on the physics of the mechanical vibration apparatus being used [4]. The MIS approach eliminates the need for approximate radiation boundary conditions by implementing a hybrid element method in which the FE method described above is used for the imaging zone and a boundary element (BE) method is used for the surrounding medium (i.e., in the breast-imaging setup, a homogeneous liquid in which the breast is immersed) [10]. The methods used to cope with boundary conditions are discussed in detail in the chapters devoted to the individual imaging modalities.

3   INVERSE PROBLEM

3.1   Gauss-Newton Iteration

The forward solution described above computes the spatial variation of an external observable (e.g., electric field) based on a given tissue-property distribution, governing equation, boundary conditions, and source terms. The *inverse* solution estimates the property distribution given the governing equation, boundary conditions, source terms, and measurements of the external observable. For all modalities considered in this book, the forward problem is linear and the inverse problem nonlinear [1, 4]. That is, the tissue properties to be estimated depend nonlinearly on the observable.

We have pursued a Gauss-Newton iterative scheme for solution of the inverse problem [1]. This approach begins with an initial estimate of the property distribution and solves the forward problem based on this initial distribution. It then compares this solution with the measured data (as specified below) and solves a linearized approximation of the inverse problem to obtain a new estimate of the property distribution. This procedure is iterative: the property-estimate updating is repeated until the algorithm converges to an optimal least-squares fit of modeled data to measured data.

We employ an iterative Newton algorithm defined by

$$\xi_{v+1} = \xi_v - \left(f'(\xi)\right)^{-1} f(\xi) \tag{2.14}$$

Here, ξ_v is the estimate of the material property distribution at the vth iteration, ξ_{v+1} is the updated estimate, and $f'(\xi)$ is the derivative of $f(\xi)$ with respect to ξ [11]. The functional $f(\xi)$ is defined in terms of a cost function, G, that expresses the difference between the measured and modeled data at each iteration:

$$G = \min \left\| \Phi(\xi) - \Phi_m \right\|^2 \tag{2.15}$$

and

$$f(\xi) = \frac{\partial G}{\partial \xi} = 2\left(\Phi(\xi) - \Phi_m\right)\frac{\partial \Phi}{\partial \xi} \tag{2.16}$$

Here, vectors $\Phi(\xi)$ and Φ_m are the computed (i.e., forward-solution) and measured values, respectively, of the observable quantity of interest at the measurement sites. Both are $O_{IM} = N_E \times O_E$ long, where N_E is the number of different excitations and O_E is the number of measurement sites per observation. (For example, in an imaging region surrounded by 16 microwave antennas, one of which transmits at any given time while the others receive, $N_E = 16$, $O_E = 15$, and $O_{IM} = 240$.) Furthermore, vectors ξ_v, ξ_{v+1}, and $\Delta\xi = \xi_{v+1} - \xi_v$ are all L long, where L is the number of material parameter values to be reconstructed. L is not necessarily equal to N, the number of nodes in the mesh used to model the observable phenomenon of interest; see discussion of the dual mesh scheme in the next section.

Using (2.16) and the fact that $f'(\xi) = 2(\partial\Phi/\partial\xi)^2$ (if $\partial^2\Phi/\partial\xi^2$ is assumed small enough to neglect),

$$\left(f'(\xi)\right)^{-1} f(\xi) = \left(\frac{\partial \Phi}{\partial \xi}\right)^{-1} \left(\Phi(\xi) - \Phi_m\right) \tag{2.17}$$

Matrix $\partial\Phi/\partial\xi$ is $(M \times O) \times L$ and is termed the Jacobian matrix, [J]. Inserting (2.17) into (2.14) and rearranging produces (in matrix notation)

$$[J]\{\Delta\xi\} = \{\Phi_m - \Phi(\xi)\} \tag{2.18}$$

where $\{\Delta\xi\} = \{\xi_{v+1}\} - \{\xi_v\}$. Multiplying both sides by $[J^T]$, we have

$$[J^T J]\{\Delta\xi\} = [J^T]\{\Phi_m - \Phi(\xi)\} \tag{2.19}$$

We wish to calculate the update vector $\{\Delta\xi\}$, which, with $\{\xi_v\}$, gives $\{\xi_{v+1}\}$ at the new iteration. The entries of $\{\Phi_m\}$ are known and the entries of $\{\Phi(\xi)\}$ are computed using $\{\xi_v\}$ by the forward-solution method described earlier. Therefore, the only term of (2.19) still needed is [J]. We obtain this by differentiating (2.12) with respect to ξ. Vector $\{b\}$ contains only boundary and forcing information; it is therefore not a function of ξ and $\{db/d\xi\} = 0$. After rearranging,

$$\left[A \right]\left[\frac{\partial\Phi}{\partial\xi} \right] = -\left[\frac{\partial A}{\partial\xi} \right]\{\Phi(\xi)\} \tag{2.20}$$

Furthermore, [A] and $\{\Phi(\xi)\}$ are computed at each iteration as part of the forward solution. Thus, only $[\partial A/\partial\xi]$ is needed to solve (2.20) for $[\partial\Phi/\partial\xi] = [J]$. The details of computing $[\partial A/\partial\xi]$ and $[\partial\Phi/\partial\xi]$ differ among the imaging modalities (see [12] and other chapters in this book). In Section 3.3, a closer look is taken at the method used for one particular modality (MIS).

A few of the computational techniques required for the efficient solution of the inverse problem will now be discussed, including the dual mesh scheme, the adjoint technique, and zone iterative reconstruction.

3.2   Dual Mesh Scheme

The system $[A]\{\Phi\} = \{b\}$ is rank N, but the dimension of the property distribution vector $\{\xi\}$ need not be N. We have exploited this fact to develop a *dual mesh* scheme [12].

In solving for the spatial distribution of the observable of interest in each modality, mesh discretization must be fine enough to meet accuracy criteria. For instance, in the MIS approach the nodes of the mesh must be separated by no more than approximately $\lambda/10$ (or one seventh of the exponential decay distance, whichever is less [13]). On the other hand, the spatial resolution required for $\{\xi\}$, which is directly related to the final image resolution, is dependent both on the spatial frequency of the parameter or parameters to be estimated (which is relatively low in all cases considered here) and on the amount of measurement data available. This points to a natural link between the amount of measurement data available and image resolution.

In the dual mesh method, the parameter ξ is represented on a mesh that is coincident with the forward-solution mesh but coarser. The nodes of this coarse mesh may be placed arbitrarily with respect to those of the mesh used for the forward solution of the observable phenomenon (Figure 4). Over each element of the L-node ("coarse" or "property") mesh, ξ is defined as a weighted sum of Lagrangian basis functions analogous to that defining $\Phi_N(x, y)$ over the N-node ("fine" or "forward-solution") mesh:

$$\xi(x,y) = \sum_{m=1}^{L} \xi_m \, \varphi_m(x,y) \qquad (2.21)$$

Each φ_m, like each ϕ_i in (2.5), is a linear basis function that is nonzero only over its associated triangular elements; however, each φ_m is associated with a node of the coarse mesh, while each ϕ_i was associated with a node of the fine mesh. The summation in (2.21), like that in (2.7), only has three nonzero terms in two dimensions (four, in three dimensions) for any (x, y) in the area covered by the mesh element.

The dual mesh approach entails some computational overhead. For instance, in solving the forward problem, the property distribution must be mapped from the parameter mesh to the forward solution mesh. However, this is a linear operation that can be accomplished efficiently by matrix multiplication. As will be seen below, more significant computational overhead occurs in calculating the terms of the Jacobian matrix, $[\partial\Phi/\partial\xi]$.

As mentioned above, computing $[\partial\Phi/\partial\xi]$ differs among modalities. For illustrative purposes, the MIS case is considered here; the following equations are therefore specifically valid only when the governing equation is (2.1). More detailed treatments for each modality are provided in other chapters.

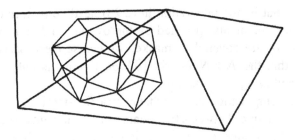

Figure 4. A portion of a parameter mesh (large triangles) with a portion of the forward-solution mesh (small triangles) that it overlays. In practice, the meshes are co-extensive.

We begin by examining the element at row i and column j of [A] in (2.12):

$$\alpha_{i,j} = \langle \nabla\phi_i \cdot \nabla\phi_j \rangle + \langle \phi_i \phi_j \xi_i \rangle \tag{2.22}$$

The first term on the right-hand side results from multiplying the divergence operator in the Helmholtz equation by the weighting function ϕ_i and applying Green's identity to produce the weak-form solution. The second term results from multiplying $\xi(x, y)$ by ϕ_j and integrating over the model domain. (In the MIS case, ξ is equal to the wave number squared, k^2.)

The next step in computing $[\partial\Phi/\partial\xi]$ is to differentiate [A] with respect to ξ_ℓ, where ℓ denotes a node in the coarse mesh. This is accomplished by differentiating (2.22). (In principle, the calculation of L derivatives of [A] is required, each an $N \times N$ matrix; however, as will be shown, only a few terms of each $[\partial A/\partial\xi_\ell]$ are nonzero.) Using the fact that neither ϕ_i nor ϕ_j is a function of ξ_ℓ and substituting for ξ_i from (2.21), differentiation of (2.22) gives

$$\frac{\partial\alpha_{i,j}}{\partial\xi_\ell} = \frac{\partial\left(\langle \nabla\phi_i \cdot \nabla\phi_j \rangle + \langle \phi_i \phi_j \xi_i \rangle\right)}{\partial\xi_\ell} = \left\langle \phi_i \phi_j \frac{\partial\xi_i}{\partial\xi_\ell} \right\rangle$$

$$= \left\langle \phi_i \phi_j \frac{\partial\left(\sum_{m=1}^{L} \xi_m \varphi_m\right)}{\partial\xi_\ell} \right\rangle = \langle \phi_i \phi_j \varphi_\ell \rangle \tag{2.23}$$

where φ_ℓ is the basis function associated with node ℓ in the parameter mesh.

Although in principle each $\langle \phi_i \phi_j \varphi_\ell \rangle$ term requires integration over the entire fine-mesh area, its argument is nonzero only where φ_ℓ, ϕ_i, and ϕ_j are all nonzero. That is, the integration in (2.23) need be performed only where those fine-mesh elements specified by the overlap of fine-mesh basis functions ϕ_i and ϕ_j are covered or masked by coarse-mesh basis function φ_ℓ. This means that the $N \times N$ matrix $[\partial A / \partial \xi_\ell]$ contains only a few nonzero elements, simplifying computation.

A minor complication arises whenever a fine-mesh element happens to straddle the boundary between two coarse-mesh elements (see Figure 3). In such a case, the argument of $\langle \phi_i \phi_j \varphi_\ell \rangle$ is nonzero over only *part* of that fine-mesh element, i.e., the part masked by φ_ℓ [12]. One might choose, when constructing the two meshes originally, to place their nodes so that each fine-mesh element resides entirely within one coarse-mesh element (no border-crossers). This would eliminate fragmentary element integrations but constrain mesh generation. Alternatively, one might allow arbitrary generation of both meshes and then perform fragmentary element integrations as needed. We have chosen the latter method [12]. The required procedures are computationally complex but not conceptually difficult.

The fact that $\partial \alpha_{i,j} / \partial \xi_\ell$ is a function only of the basis functions of the fine and coarse meshes offers large computational savings. Since the basis functions are a fixed feature of algorithm design, all nonzero elements of $[\partial A / \partial \xi_\ell]$ can be precalculated and stored in a lookup table, which saves the effort of recomputing them at each iteration.

3.3   Adjoint Method

A direct-differentiation technique for constructing the Jacobian matrix, which is used to solve for the property update vector $\{\Delta \xi\}$ at each iteration, was described in Section 3.1. However, this method can be computationally expensive. For instance, in a case where the forward-solution and parameter meshes have N and L nodes, respectively, and are surrounded by N_E source excitations, the computational load at each iteration includes (a) N_E LU factorizations of [A] and N_E matrix back-substitutions for the forward problem and (b) $N_E \times L$ matrix back-substitutions for the inverse problem.

Little can be done to reduce the computational costs of the forward problem. However, in the inverse problem an alternative to direct computation of the Jacobian matrix is the *adjoint method* [14]. This is utilized in the NIS, EIS, and MIS modalities, where the principle of reciprocity can be exploited. Reciprocity holds where, for a fixed property distribution, the physical phenomenon measured at point r due to a given source at point s is equal to that which would be measured at s due to an equivalent source at r [15].

Interchangeability of image and source in lens optics is an example of reciprocity.

Each entry of the Jacobian matrix describes the change in the observable (e.g., electromagnetic field) corresponding to an infinitesimal property change at node ℓ in the coarse mesh, where the wave phenomenon is generated by a point source at location s and is measured at location r. Each entry in the Jacobian can thus be written as

$$J_{s,r,\ell} = \left\langle \frac{\partial \Phi_s}{\partial \xi_\ell} \delta(x_r, y_r) \right\rangle \tag{2.24}$$

where Φ_s is the distribution of the observable resulting from a point source at s, δ is the Dirac delta function, x_r and y_r are the Cartesian coordinates of the measurement site r, and $\langle \cdot \rangle$ signifies integration over the region where φ_ℓ, the coarse-mesh basis function at node ℓ, is nonzero. Putting (2.24) aside for the moment, we rewrite (2.20) as

$$\left[A \right] \left[\frac{\partial \Phi_s}{\partial \xi_\ell} \right] = -\left[\frac{\partial A}{\partial \xi_\ell} \right] \{\Phi_s\} = \{b_{eff}\} \tag{2.25}$$

Here, the right-hand side has been set equal to $\{b_{eff}\}$, an "effective" source; that is, $\{b_{eff}\}$ holds the same place in (2.25) as does the source term $\{b\}$ in (2.12).

By reciprocity, if an auxiliary source $\{b_r\}$ is (conceptually) placed at the receiver location r, the resulting observable $\{\Phi_r\}$ is found by solving

$$[A]\{\Phi_r\} = \{b_r\} \tag{2.26}$$

Here, each of the N entries of $\{b_r\}$ is given by the inner product $\langle \phi_i V_r \rangle$, which is constructed by the process described in Section 2.2 (i.e., ϕ_i is the ith forward-mesh basis function employed as a weighting function). In agreement with assumption in (2.24) of a point source, V_r is chosen as

$$V_r = |V_r| \delta(x_r, y_r) \tag{2.27}$$

Combining (2.25) and (2.26) by reciprocity (and temporarily dropping matrix notation for simplicity), we obtain

$$\left\langle b_r \frac{\partial \Phi_s}{\partial \xi_\ell} \right\rangle = \left\langle b_{\mathit{eff}} \Phi_r \right\rangle \tag{2.28}$$

By (2.25), $b_{\mathit{eff}} = -(\partial A/\partial \xi_\ell)\Phi_s$, where the (i, j)th element of $\partial A/\partial \xi_\ell$ is (as shown in the previous section) given by $\langle \phi_i \phi_j \varphi_\ell \rangle$. Substituting for terms on both sides of (2.28) thus yields, for a reciprocal point source b_r,

$$\left\langle |V_r| \delta(x_r, y_r) \frac{\partial \Phi_s}{\partial \xi_\ell} \right\rangle = -\left\langle \left\langle \phi_i \phi_j \varphi_\ell \right\rangle \Phi_r \Phi_s \right\rangle \tag{2.29}$$

Dividing both sides of (2.29) by $|V_r|$ produces

$$\left\langle \frac{\partial \Phi_s}{\partial \xi_\ell} \delta(x_r, y_r) \right\rangle = -\frac{1}{|V_r|} \left\langle \left\langle \phi_i \phi_j \varphi_\ell \right\rangle \Phi_r \Phi_s \right\rangle \tag{2.30}$$

The left-hand term, per (2.24), is $J_{s,r,\ell}$. Since all values of $\langle \phi_i \phi_j \varphi_\ell \rangle$ can be stored as a precomputed weighting vector, each entry of the Jacobian can be computed during image reconstruction by means of a simple inner product of $\langle \Phi_s \Phi_r \rangle$ times a constant (i.e., $\langle \phi_i \phi_j \varphi_\ell \rangle / |V_r|$)—always providing that the sources and receivers are colocated, i.e., that each source antenna can also be configured to operate as a receiver. (In practice, many $J_{s,r,\ell}$ need not be computed because $\langle \phi_i \phi_j \varphi_\ell \rangle$ is often zero.) This computation is an $O(N)$ operation, in contrast to the $O(N \times M)$ matrix back-substitutions in (2.20), where M is the bandwidth of the sparse matrix $[A]$. For large N, the savings can be significant. Finally, this approach is quite general and can be readily expanded to 3D for each modality.

3.4   Iterative Reconstruction in MRE

In the MRE system, tissue is vibrated along a single axis at low amplitude and low frequency. This excitation is phase-locked to the sequencing of the MR system to measure the harmonic displacement of each pixel in space. Because an information-rich volumetric data set is acquired in this case, strategies other than those described above (which exploit the fact that there are relatively few observations) must be utilized to improve computational efficiency. In the MRE case, the volumetric nature of the data allows dissection of the problem into multiple subzones, where the boundary conditions of each subzone are essentially the MR-measured displacements at each boundary node. Coupling of these multiple subzone problems allows for accurate and efficient calculation of the inverse problem. The details of this approach are covered in Chapter 3, Sections 3–5.

4   ILL-CONDITIONING OF THE INVERSE PROBLEM

In all the approaches described above, the inverse problem is ill-conditioned. That is, the iterative procedure defined in (2.14)–(2.20) may not converge to a useful solution without the placement of additional restrictions on the process [16].

One way to assess ill-conditioning is to calculate the *condition number* of the Jacobian matrix, that is, the ratio of the largest eigenvalue of the system to the smallest [8]. As the condition number approaches or exceeds the numerical accuracy of the computer to be used, the system of equations is said to be unstable and the likelihood that the algorithm will converge diminishes. In effect, the system of equations is rank deficient and the amount of independent measurement information is not adequate.

Before discussing some of the standard mathematical approaches to ill-conditioning, it should be said that certain strategies can mitigate the problem without applying regularization methods. In general, adding more measurement data will improve the process, but it is not always clear how linearly independent the new data will be compared to the existing measurement set. In addition, the cost of adding new receiver channels can be high. Unwanted source and receiver interactions could be exacerbated by placing more receivers in an already crowded volume [17], and the added computational costs may be significant. However, there are important opportunities here. For instance, in all three tomographic approaches, data are acquired at multiple frequencies. Preliminary eigenvalue studies with the MIS system suggest that the inclusion of additional multifrequency data reduces the system condition number. Interestingly, depending on the individual system and on the orientation of sources and receivers, certain data (e.g., signals passing directly through the tissue versus signals diffracted to the sides) are clearly more valuable than others [18]. Finally, the problem statement itself can have a significant effect on the condition number. For instance, in the MIS system the eigenvalue spectral content is significantly improved when the minimization statement (2.15) starts from the log magnitude and phase form of the electric-field values rather than the more traditional complex form [18]. It has been shown that the former emphasizes the directly-transmitted data over the signals received by antennas close to the transmitter, and that the opposite is the case for the complex-form algorithm. Attention to features other than regularization can thus be important.

4.1   Tikhonov Regularization

The most common approach to regularization is the Tikhonov method [16]. This approach begins with the minimization statement given in (2.15) and adds a weighted penalty term:

$$G = \min \left\| \Phi(\xi) - \Phi_m \right\|^2 + \rho \left\| \xi - \xi^* \right\|^2 \qquad (2.31)$$

In this case, the penalized factor is a Euclidean distance term referenced to ξ^* with ρ as the weight. Other forms incorporate the first or second derivative of the property distribution. Now, $f(\xi)$ and its derivative $f'(\xi)$, referred to by (2.14), are given by

$$f(\xi) = \frac{\partial G}{\partial \xi} = 2\left(\Phi(\xi) - \Phi_m \right) \frac{\partial \Phi}{\partial \xi} + 2\rho\left(\xi - \xi^* \right) \qquad (2.32)$$

and
$$f'(\xi) = 2 \frac{\partial \Phi}{\partial \xi} \frac{\partial \Phi}{\partial \xi} + 2\rho \qquad (2.33)$$

where the second-order derivative of $\Phi(\xi)$ is ignored in determining $f'(\theta)$. Combining (2.14) and (2.33) yields

$$\Delta\xi = \left(\frac{\partial \Phi}{\partial \xi} \frac{\partial \Phi}{\partial \xi} + \rho \right)^{-1} \left[\frac{\partial \Phi}{\partial \xi} \left(\Phi_m - \Phi(\xi) \right) - \rho\left(\xi - \xi^* \right) \right] \qquad (2.34)$$

This can be rewritten in matrix form as

$$\left[J^T J + \rho I \right] \{ \Delta\xi \} = \left[J^T \right] \{ \Phi_m - \Phi(\xi) \} - \rho\{ \xi - \xi^* \} \qquad (2.35)$$

where $[J] = [\partial\Phi/\partial\xi]$, $[I]$ is the $N \times N$ identity matrix, and ξ denotes the property values at iteration i.

The value of ξ^* is usually fixed. However, in one variation of this procedure, ξ^* is set equal to the parameter distribution at the previous iteration, ξ_i. This variation is termed the Levenberg-Marquardt algorithm [1, 19, 20]. In this case, (2.35) simplifies to

$$\left[J^T J + 2\rho I\right]\left\{\Delta\xi\right\} = \left[J^T\right]\left\{\Phi_m - \Phi(\xi)\right\} \tag{2.36}$$

This method is of interest because it removes the penalty term from the gradient (i.e., the right-hand side of the equation).

In general, the convergence characteristics of the two approaches (i.e., conventional, as in (2.14)–(2.20), versus with Tikhonov regularization) are distinct and problem-specific [10, 21].

4.2   Hessian Scaling and Tikhonov Weight

The net effect of the regularization on the Hessian matrix $[J^T J]$ is to ensure its diagonal dominance, which facilitates its LU factorization [8]. However, determining the optimal weighting factor ρ is problem-specific and can be quite difficult [22, 23]. One complication is that the scale of the elements of the Hessian matrix can vary considerably from one imaging session to the next. A novel approach was developed by Joachimowicz and colleagues [21], who set ρ equal to the trace of the Hessian matrix multiplied by an empirically determined factor, α, and the relative least-square error at each iteration, e_{rel}:

$$\rho = \alpha\, e_{rel}\, \text{trace}\left(\left[J^T J\right]\right) \tag{2.37}$$

Reducing the net regularization parameter as the iterations progress allows the influence of the less-dominant eigenvalues to be gradually introduced. That is, with large ρ at the algorithm's start, a blurred or smooth image is initially reconstructed; as ρ is reduced at each iteration, more detail appears (but the solution edges toward instability). The trace essentially measures the scaling effect of the matrix $[A]$ on the vector $\{\Phi\}$ in (2.12) [8]. Therefore, the level of regularization can be controlled (to some degree) by the dimensionless quantity ρ.

One consequence of this approach is that since the Hessian diagonal terms can vary in magnitude, the influence of the regularization is uneven across the span of reconstruction parameters. Marquardt [20] introduced a matrix scaling (previously associated with the Levenberg regularization technique) that normalizes all Hessian diagonal terms to unity [19, 20]. Multiplying both sides of (2.18) by a diagonal matrix $[G]$ and inserting the identity matrix (written as $[GG^{-1}]$) between the Hessian matrix $[J^T J]$ and the update vector $\{\Delta\xi\}$, we have

$$\left[\, G \,\right]\!\left[J^T J \right]\!\left[G G^{-1} \right]\!\{\Delta\xi\} = \left[\, G \,\right]\!\left[J^T \right]\!\{\Phi^m - \Phi^c\} \tag{2.38}$$

which can be rewritten as

$$\left[G J^T J G \right]\!\left\{\left[G^{-1} \right]\!\{\Delta\xi\}\right\} = \left[G J^T \right]\!\{\Phi^m - \Phi^c\} \tag{2.39}$$

and solved for $\{[G^{-1}]\{\Delta\xi\}\}$, which we will call $\{\Delta\xi\}^*$. (Note that $\{\Delta\xi\}$ itself can be easily recovered from $\{\Delta\xi\}^*$, as $[G]$ is diagonal.) The nonzero elements of $[G]$ are chosen as

$$g_{ii} = \frac{1}{\sqrt{h_{ii}}} \tag{2.40}$$

where g_{ii} and h_{ii} are the diagonal elements of $[G]$ and of the Hessian matrix $[J^T J]$, respectively. All diagonal entries of the scaled Hessian matrix $[GJ^T JG]$ are unity, allowing for the level of regularization to be controlled by the addition to the diagonal of a single nondimensional quantity (e.g., λ). This quantity can be empirically chosen so that the algorithm is relatively robust across a broad span of imaging tasks.

4.3   Miscellaneous Techniques

We have utilized two additional techniques which generally act as forms of regularization. The first is a spatial filtering approach. When the property distribution is updated at each iteration, uneven fluctuations in the intermediate image can occur, especially during the early stages of the process. We have devised a spatial filter which can be applied through a matrix-vector multiplication that forms a weighted average of the value at node i with those of its surrounding neighbors [24]:

$$\xi_i^{new} = q\,\xi_i^{old} + \frac{(1-q)}{T}\sum_{j=1}^{T}\xi_j^{old} \tag{2.41}$$

Here, q is chosen to be between 0 and 1, T is the number of nodes to be averaged, and the superscripts "old" and "new" refer to the property values before and after application of the filter, respectively. As q varies from 1 to 0, the amount of filtering goes from none to full averaging with the T neighboring values.

Another technique is to reduce the iteration step size [25, 26]. Modifying (2.14) slightly produces

$$\{\xi\}_{i+1} = \{\xi\}_i + \tau\{\Delta\xi\} \tag{2.42}$$

where τ, which may be varied from 0 to 1, controls the step size.

It has been noted that in Newton iterative techniques, the computed update values can overshoot the desired values by a considerable margin, especially when the starting property distribution is not chosen carefully [11]. Reducing the step size may slow convergence, but is another useful tool for stabilizing an inherently unstable process.

5   3D IMAGING

In all of the imaging modalities discussed here, the physics of the electromagnetic wave propagation or mechanical vibration are intrinsically three-dimensional. To achieve 3D images is a sizeable computational task, especially given limitations on data acquisition and computational resources. Within each modality, therefore, we performed experiments to assess the image degradation to be expected from using approximate 2D algorithms. Results varied by modality. In MRE, it was found that a 2D approach was inadequate, while in MIS it was shown that 3D effects were greatly reduced by utilizing a low-contrast coupling medium (i.e., choosing a fluid bath with electrical properties as close as possible to those of the breast [27]).

In all four modalities, the ultimate goal is full 3D imaging. This can be achieved by incrementally perfecting tools for the 2D and 2.5D (hybrid of 2D and 3D) cases, and by designing these tools to be generalizable to fully 3D approaches. For example, the FE methods associated with the forward and inverse problems outlined in this chapter can be straightforwardly, albeit with effort, generalized to 3D. The degree to which 3D implementations are being explored for each modality is briefly discussed in the ensuing modality chapters.

6   CONCLUSION

This chapter has provided a brief overview of the iterative approach utilized in some form by all four imaging modalities treated in this book. It has outlined the basic notions of the inverse problem and highlighted issues such as computational cost and ill-conditioning. The dual mesh scheme, adjoint method, and regularization strategies have been discussed, along with their implications for the imaging process. The methods outlined here are, however, by no means exhaustive or final.

The breast is a particularly intriguing imaging target for all four modalities because of its accessibility and relatively small volume. The complexity of the data acquisition systems required is not overly burdensome and the resources needed, even for the computationally intensive algorithms outlined here, are within reach.

REFERENCES

[1]   B. Kaltenbacher, "Newton-type methods for ill-posed problems." *Inverse Probl.*, Vol. 13, 1997, pp. 729–753.

[2]   A. Papoulis, *The Fourier Integral and Its Applications* (New York: McGraw-Hill, 1962).

[3]   R. F. Harrington, *Field Computation by Moment Methods* (Melbourne, FL: R. E. Krieger Publishing Co., 1968).

[4]   J. N. Reddy, *An Introduction to the Finite Element Method*, 2nd Ed. (New York: McGraw-Hill, 1993).

[5]   G. D. Smith, *Numerical Solution of Partial Differential Equations: Finite Difference Method* (Oxford: Clarendon Press, 1985).

[6]   A. Taflove and S. Hagness, *Computational Electrodynamics: The Finite-Difference Time-Domain Method*, 2nd Ed. (Boston: Artech House, 2000).

[7]   K. D. Paulsen and W. Liu, "Memory and operations count scaling for coupled finite element and boundary element systems of equations." *Int. J. Numerical Methods in Eng.*, Vol. 33, 1992, pp. 1289–1304.

[8]   G. H. Golub and C. F. van Loan, *Matrix Computations*, 2nd Ed. (Baltimore, MD: Johns Hopkins Univ. Press, 1989).

[9]   T. B. A. Senior and J. L. Volakis, *Approximate Boundary Conditions in Electromagnetics* (London: Institution of Electrical Engineers, 1995).

[10]   P. M. Meaney, K. D. Paulsen, and T. P. Ryan, "Two-dimensional hybrid element image reconstruction for TM illumination." *IEEE Trans. Ant. and Prop.*, Vol. 43, 1995, pp. 239–247.

[11]   J. H. Mathews, *Numerical Methods for Mathematics, Science, and Engineering* (Englewood, NJ: Prentice-Hall, 1992).

[12]   K. D. Paulsen et al., "A dual mesh scheme for finite element based reconstruction algorithms." *IEEE Trans. Med. Imag.*, Vol. 14, 1995, pp. 504–514.

[13]   D. R. Lynch, K. D. Paulsen, and J. W. Strohbehn, "Finite element solution of Maxwell's equations for hyperthermic treatment planning." *J. Computational Physics*, Vol. 58(2), 1985, pp. 246–249.

[14]   Q. Fang et al., "Microwave image reconstruction from 3D fields coupled to 2D parameter estimation." *IEEE Trans. Med. Imag.*, 2004 (accepted).

[15]   P. M. Meaney, N. K. Yagnamurthy, and K. D. Paulsen, "Pre-scaling of reconstruction parameter components to reduce imbalance in image recovery process." *Physics Med. Biol.*, Vol. 47, 2002, pp. 1101–1119.

[16]   A. N. Tikhonov and V. Y. Arsenin, *Solutions of Ill-Posed Problems* (Washington, D.C.: Winston, 1977).

[17] D. M. Pozar and D. H. Schaubert, *Microstrip Antennas: The Analysis of Microstrip Antennas and Arrays* (New York: Wiley-IEEE Press, 2001).

[18] P. M. Meaney et al., "Microwave image reconstruction utilizing log-magnitude and un-wrapped phase to improve high-contrast object recovery." *IEEE Trans. Med. Imag.*, Vol. 20, 2001, pp. 104–116.

[19] K. Levenberg, "A Method for the solution of certain nonlinear problems in least squares." *Q. Appl. Math.*, Vol. 2, 1944, pp. 164–168.

[20] D. W. Marquardt, "An algorithm for least-squares estimation of nonlinear parameters." *J. Soc. Ind. Appl. Math.*, Vol. 11, 1963, pp. 431–441.

[21] N. Joachimowicz, C. Pichot, and J. R. Hugonin, "Inverse scattering: An iterative numerical method for electromagnetic imaging." *IEEE Trans. Antennas Propagat.*, Vol. 39, 1991, pp. 1742–1752.

[22] P. M. Meaney et al., "A two-stage microwave image reconstruction procedure for improved internal feature extraction." *Med. Phys.*, Vol. 28, 2001, pp. 2358–2369.

[23] D. Calvetti et al., "Tikhonov regularization and the L-curve for large discrete ill-posed problems." *J. Comput. Appl. Math.*, Vol. 123, 2000, pp. 423–446.

[24] P. M. Meaney et al., "A two-stage microwave image reconstruction procedure for improved internal feature extraction." *Med. Phys.*, Vol. 28, 2001, pp. 2358–2369.

[25] D. M. Bates and D. G. Watts, *Nonlinear Regression and Its Applications* (New York: Wiley, 1988).

[26] G. F. F. Seber and C. J. Wild, *Nonlinear Regression* (New York: Wiley, 1989).

[27] P. M. Meaney et al., "Importance of using a reduced-contrast coupling medium in 2D microwave breast imaging." *Int. J. Hyperthermia*, Vol. 19, 2003, pp. 534–550.

Chapter 3

MAGNETIC RESONANCE ELASTOGRAPHY: THEORY

Elijah E. W. Van Houten, Ph.D. and Marvin Doyley, Ph.D.

1   INTRODUCTION

Model-based mechanical property imaging is achieved by applying mechanical energy to a target object (e.g., the breast), measuring the target's response, and using these measurements to optimize a numerical model of the distribution of some mechanical property or properties throughout the object. In the method discussed in this chapter, magnetic resonance elastography (MRE), low-frequency vibrations are applied to the target and spatial displacements are measured within it by means of phase-contrast magnetic resonance imaging (MRI). Harmonic displacements within the domain of interest are measured in phase with the mechanical excitation and compared to displacements calculated using a numerical model of the elastic-property distribution within the target volume. The model property distribution is then iteratively adjusted until its predictions converge with observation. An image is generated from the final model property distribution.

Other elasticity imaging methods are being developed. Perhaps the most common alternative to reconstruction-based (model-based) elasticity imaging is the conversion of displacement measurements into strain values, which can in turn be used to solve directly for elastic property values [1, 2]. Other approaches to reconstructive elasticity imaging compare measured strains and their resultant stresses [3]. Elastography methods can also be classified according to the method of mechanical excitation employed; some methods use harmonic or wavefront excitation [1, 2, 4], while others use quasistatic excitation [5].

2   RECONSTRUCTIVE ELASTICITY IMAGING

The model used to relate the current property estimate to the observable data is a key component of any reconstructive imaging method. The equations of linear elasticity, which relate stress to strain via an elastic modulus, are an obvious choice for the governing equations of motion in our elastographic imaging method.

2.1   Equations of Linear Elasticity

The most basic relations of solid mechanics are the equations of linear elasticity. These assume a linear relationship between stress (applied pressure) and strain (material deformation), an approximation valid for most materials when strain levels are low. The relative simplicity of the equations of linear elasticity makes them a popular estimator even when dealing with mildly nonlinear materials or moderately high strain. Their full derivation is beyond the scope of this work, but the interested reader is directed to the excellent text by Chou and Pagano [6]. A brief summary is given here.

A *stress*, σ, applied to a deformable material, causes a deformation or *strain*, ε. On the surface of an infinitesimal cube one can define three normal stresses σ_i (i.e., pressures normal to the surfaces of the cube, each σ_i aligned with the ith spatial dimension) and six shear stresses σ_{ij}, $i \neq j$ (i.e., pressures acting along the jth dimension and normal to the ith dimension). For an infinitesimal cube, only three of the shear stress terms σ_{ij} are independent, so altogether only six stress terms are considered. These six terms — σ_1, σ_2, σ_3, σ_{12}, σ_{13}, and σ_{23} — constitute the *symmetric stress tensor*. Similarly, the *symmetric strain tensor* comprises three normal strain terms ε_i and three independent shearing strain terms ε_{ij}. Each normal strain ε_i is defined in terms of the displacement u_i of a surface of the infinitesimal cube along the ith dimension x_i, i.e.,

$$\varepsilon_i = \frac{\partial u_i}{\partial x_i} \tag{3.1}$$

Each shearing strain ε_{ij} is given by

$$\varepsilon_{ij} = \frac{1}{2}\left(\frac{\partial u_i}{\partial x_j} + \frac{\partial u_j}{\partial x_i}\right) \text{ for } i \neq j. \qquad (3.2)$$

The displacements u_i at a point constitute the *displacement field* at that point.

For linearly elastic materials, the relationship between the stress tensor and the strain tensor is given by Hooke's law:

$$\{\sigma\} = [C]\{\varepsilon\} \qquad (3.3)$$

[C] is termed the *material matrix* or *modulus matrix* and has entries that are simple functions of two constants, namely, Young's modulus, E, and Poisson's ratio, v.

Hooke's law (3.3) can be used to formulate a governing equation for a time-varying displacement field by invoking Newton's third law in terms of stress and displacement:

$$\frac{\partial \sigma_{ij}}{\partial x_i} + F_i = \rho \frac{\partial^2 u_i}{\partial t^2} \qquad (3.4)$$

Here, x_i is the ith spatial coordinate; F_i and u_i are body force and displacement, respectively, along the ith direction (a *body force* being a force distributed throughout a body's volume, e.g., gravitational force); t is time; and ρ is density. Reformulation of (3.4) leads to the partial differential equation commonly known as Navier's equation:

$$\nabla \cdot \mu \nabla \mathbf{u} + \nabla(\lambda + \mu)\nabla \cdot \mathbf{u} = \rho \frac{\partial^2 \mathbf{u}}{\partial t^2} \qquad (3.5)$$

Here $\mathbf{u}$ is vector displacement and μ and λ are the material stiffness moduli known as Lamé's constants, which are related to Young's modulus and Poisson's ratio by

$$\lambda = \frac{Ev}{(1+v)(1-2v)} \qquad (3.6)$$

and
$$\mu = \frac{E}{2(1+v)} \qquad (3.7)$$

A system of linear algebraic equations whose solution specifies an approximation to **u** in (3.5) is obtained using the method of weighted residuals, as described in detail in Ch. 2, Sec. 2.2. This system of equations is discussed in the following section.

2.2   Discretized Formulation of Reconstructive Elasticity Imaging Problem

Reconstructive imaging involves a set of measurements, y, a parameter image, θ, and a numerical or analytic model, $f(\theta)$, that relates y to θ. Given y, $f(\theta)$ allows estimation of a parameter image θ; given θ, it allows generation of a set of simulated measurements $\hat{y} = f(\theta)$. (See Ch. 2 for fuller discussion of iterative reconstructive imaging.) Some method for solving $f(\theta)$ over task-appropriate geometries is also required.

In our case, Navier's equation (3.5) lends itself to analytic solution for only the simplest geometries and material property descriptions. This necessitates a numerical approach. The long association of the finite element (FE) method with problems in linear elasticity makes it an obvious choice for solving a discretized formulation of (3.5). Our $f(\theta)$ is, therefore, a finite element model based on (3.5) and covering the imaging zone. (Note that in MRE, unlike the other three modalities covered in this book, the reconstruction parameter mesh is the same as the forward solution mesh, due to the fact that displacement measurement data are given for each node by MR.)

Using the FE weighted-residual method on a three-dimensional mesh with N_N nodes, (3.5) can be rewritten for an approximate displacement field $\{\hat{u}\}$ as

$$\left[A(\mu,\lambda,\rho)\right]\{\hat{u}\} = \{b\} \qquad (3.8)$$

Here $\{\hat{u}\}$ has $3N_N$ entries, $\{b\}$ is a vector of forcing (source) terms having $3N_N$ entries, and $[A(\mu,\lambda,\rho)]$ is $3N_N \times 3N_N$ and has the form

$$\left[A_{ij}\right] = \begin{bmatrix} a_{11} & a_{12} & a_{13} \\ a_{21} & a_{22} & a_{23} \\ a_{31} & a_{32} & a_{33} \end{bmatrix} \qquad (3.9)$$

for any i,j combination, where

$$a_{11} = \left\langle \frac{\partial \phi_i}{\partial x}\frac{\partial \phi_j}{\partial x}\left(2S_\mu + S_\lambda\right) + \frac{\partial \phi_i}{\partial y}\frac{\partial \phi_j}{\partial y}S_\mu + \frac{\partial \phi_i}{\partial z}\frac{\partial \phi_j}{\partial z}S_\mu - \omega^2 \phi_i \phi_j S_\rho \right\rangle,$$

$$a_{12} = \left\langle \frac{\partial \phi_i}{\partial x}\frac{\partial \phi_j}{\partial y}S_\lambda + \frac{\partial \phi_i}{\partial y}\frac{\partial \phi_j}{\partial x}S_\mu \right\rangle, \quad a_{13} = \left\langle \frac{\partial \phi_i}{\partial x}\frac{\partial \phi_j}{\partial z}S_\lambda + \frac{\partial \phi_i}{\partial z}\frac{\partial \phi_j}{\partial x}S_\mu \right\rangle,$$

$$a_{21} = \left\langle \frac{\partial \phi_i}{\partial y}\frac{\partial \phi_j}{\partial x}S_\lambda + \frac{\partial \phi_i}{\partial x}\frac{\partial \phi_j}{\partial y}S_\mu \right\rangle, \quad a_{23} = \left\langle \frac{\partial \phi_i}{\partial y}\frac{\partial \phi_j}{\partial z}S_\lambda + \frac{\partial \phi_i}{\partial z}\frac{\partial \phi_j}{\partial y}S_\mu \right\rangle,$$

$$a_{22} = \left\langle \frac{\partial \phi_i}{\partial x}\frac{\partial \phi_j}{\partial x}S_\mu + \frac{\partial \phi_i}{\partial y}\frac{\partial \phi_j}{\partial y}\left(2S_\mu + S_\lambda\right) + \frac{\partial \phi_i}{\partial z}\frac{\partial \phi_j}{\partial z}S_\mu - \omega^2 \phi_i \phi_j S_\rho \right\rangle,$$

$$a_{31} = \left\langle \frac{\partial \phi_i}{\partial z}\frac{\partial \phi_j}{\partial x}S_\lambda + \frac{\partial \phi_i}{\partial x}\frac{\partial \phi_j}{\partial z}S_\mu \right\rangle, \quad a_{32} = \left\langle \frac{\partial \phi_i}{\partial z}\frac{\partial \phi_j}{\partial y}S_\lambda + \frac{\partial \phi_i}{\partial y}\frac{\partial \phi_j}{\partial z}S_\mu \right\rangle,$$

and $\quad a_{33} = \left\langle \frac{\partial \phi_i}{\partial x}\frac{\partial \phi_j}{\partial x}S_\mu + \frac{\partial \phi_i}{\partial y}\frac{\partial \phi_j}{\partial y}S_\mu + \frac{\partial \phi_i}{\partial z}\frac{\partial \phi_j}{\partial z}\left(2S_\mu + S_\lambda\right) - \omega^2 \phi_i \phi_j S_\rho \right\rangle.$

Here, each ϕ_x is a piecewise-linear Lagrangian basis function defined on the FE mesh as described in Chapter 2, i is the row index, j is the column index, and

$$S_\mu = \sum_{k=1}^{N_N} \mu_k \phi_k, \quad S_\lambda = \sum_{k=1}^{N_N} \lambda_k \phi_k, \quad \text{and} \quad S_\rho = \sum_{k=1}^{N_N} \rho_k \phi_k \qquad (3.10)$$

It is assumed that the displacement field has the time-harmonic form $\mathbf{u}(x,y,z,t) = \text{Re}\{\bar{\mathbf{u}}(x,y,z)e^{i\omega t}\}$.

To iteratively update the parameter set θ in accordance with

$$[J^T J]\{\Delta \theta\} = [J^T]\{f_m - f(\theta)\} \qquad (3.11)$$

the Jacobian matrix, $J = [\partial f / \partial \theta]$, must be computed.[*] In terms of the FE discretized linear elasticity equations, $f(\theta)$ is the calculated displacement solution, $\{\hat{\mathbf{u}}\}$, from (3.8) (sometimes termed the "forward solution") and θ stands for one of the three parameters μ, λ, or ρ.

---

[*] (3.11) was given in Ch. 2 as (2.19), where $\Phi(\xi)$ was used instead of $f(\theta)$.

The first step in determining the entries of $[\partial f/\partial\theta]$ is to differentiate (3.5) with respect to θ_k, that is, with respect to the value of μ, λ, or ρ at node k of the FE parameter mesh covering the imaging region:

$$\nabla\cdot\frac{\partial\mu}{\partial\theta_k}\nabla\mathbf{u}+\nabla\cdot\mu\nabla\frac{\partial\mathbf{u}}{\partial\theta_k}+\nabla\frac{\partial(\lambda+\mu)}{\partial\theta_k}\nabla\cdot\mathbf{u}+\nabla(\lambda+\mu)\nabla\cdot\frac{\partial\mathbf{u}}{\partial\theta_k}$$

$$=\frac{\partial\rho}{\partial\theta_k}\frac{\partial^2\mathbf{u}}{\partial t^2}+\rho\frac{\partial^3\mathbf{u}}{\partial t^2\partial\theta_k}$$

(3.12)

or $\nabla\cdot\mu\nabla\mathbf{u}'_k+\nabla(\lambda+\mu)\nabla\cdot\mathbf{u}'_k=\rho\dfrac{\partial^2\mathbf{u}'_k}{\partial t^2}+\dfrac{\partial\rho}{\partial\theta_k}\dfrac{\partial^2\mathbf{u}}{\partial t^2}$

$$-\nabla\cdot\frac{\partial\mu}{\partial\theta_k}\nabla\mathbf{u}-\nabla\frac{\partial(\lambda+\mu)}{\partial\theta_k}\nabla\cdot\mathbf{u}$$

(3.13)

This is formally identical to (3.5), except that $\mathbf{u}'_k=\partial\mathbf{u}/\partial\theta_k$ takes the place of $\mathbf{u}$ and there are two additional quantities on the right-hand side. Since (3.11) is evaluated for the current property estimate θ and the source or forcing vector $\{b\}$ is known, (3.8) can be solved for $\mathbf{u}$; this leaves $\mathbf{u}'_k$ the only unknown in (3.13), which can be solved by FE weighted-residuals discretization in the same manner as (3.5), formally yielding

$$\left\{\frac{\partial\hat{\mathbf{u}}}{\partial\theta_k}\right\}=\left[\ A\ \right]^{-1}\left\{\left[\frac{\partial A}{\partial\theta_k}\right]\{\hat{\mathbf{u}}\}\right\}$$

(3.14)

where $[A]$ and $[\partial A/\partial\theta_k]$ are $3N_N\times3N_N$ and all of the vectors are length $3N_N$. Here, the matrix $[\partial A/\partial\theta_k]$ consists of the weighted-residual entries generated by the terms involving $\mathbf{u}$ appearing in the right-hand side of (3.13). Its elements are derived from the submatrices specified by (3.10), and their evaluation depends on whether θ_k represents μ_k, λ_k, or ρ_k. For example, $\partial a_{11}/\partial\theta_k$ is

$$\frac{\partial a_{11}}{\partial\mu_k}=\left\langle\theta_k\left(2\frac{\partial\phi_i}{\partial x}\frac{\partial\phi_j}{\partial x}+\frac{\partial\phi_i}{\partial y}\frac{\partial\phi_j}{\partial y}+\frac{\partial\phi_i}{\partial z}\frac{\partial\phi_j}{\partial z}\right)\right\rangle\ \text{for}\ \theta_k=\mu_k,$$

$$\frac{\partial a_{11}}{\partial\lambda_k}=\left\langle\theta_k\frac{\partial\phi_i}{\partial x}\frac{\partial\phi_j}{\partial x}\right\rangle\ \text{for}\ \theta_k=\lambda_k,\ \text{and}$$

$$\frac{\partial a_{11}}{\partial\rho_k}=\left\langle-\phi_k\omega^2\phi_i\phi_j\right\rangle\ \text{for}\ \theta_k=\rho_k.$$

(3.15)

Finally, the Jacobian matrix, $[\partial f/\partial\theta]$, is assembled column by column from the vectors $\{\partial\hat{u}/\partial\theta_k\}$, which involve re-solution of (3.14). The approximate Hessian matrix $[J^TJ] = [\partial f/\partial\theta]^T[\partial f/\partial\theta]$ is then generated by direct matrix multiplication and (3.11) is solved for the updated parameter vector.

3   SUBZONE-BASED RECONSTRUCTION ALGORITHM FOR MRE

One might expect that the availability of full-volume, pixel-resolution displacement data from the motion-encoding gradients would automatically make a high-resolution parameter image achievable; however, the computational burden of generating iterative updates for the large number of voxels in an MR data set is too large even for today's processors. For example, a typical MRI displacement map consists of 16 image slices, each discretized to 256×256 data points. A single property data set thus has 1,048,576 measurement entries, which is several orders of magnitude more than a typical data set from any of the other modalities discussed in this book. Further, the approximate Hessian $[J^TJ]$ is generally a full matrix whose inversion requires $O(N_P^3)$ floating-point operations. Generation of the Hessian would, therefore, entail $O(10^{14})$ to $O(10^{18})$ floating-point operations and its inversion $O(10^{18})$ floating-point operations. Hence, some type of rescaling is required for successful reconstructive error minimization in order to estimate property distributions at such high resolution.

An approach that capitalizes on the data-rich environment provided by MR measurement acquisition while remaining computationally tractable is the subzone-based method for property reconstruction [4]. This technique breaks down the global minimization problem so that the functional to be minimized is distributed onto Q subzones, that is,

$$F(\theta) = \sum_{z=1}^{Q} F_z(\theta_z) \tag{3.16}$$

where θ_z is the nodal parameter distribution within the region of subzone z. The minimization of $F(\theta)$ is then carried out under the assumption that the minimization of the sum of subzones is equivalent to the sum of minimizations of each subzone:

$$\min_{\theta}\big(F(\theta)\big) \approx \min_{\theta_z}\bigg(\sum_{z=1}^{Q} F_z(\theta)\bigg) \approx \sum_{z=1}^{Q} \min_{\theta_z}\big(F_z(\theta)\big) \tag{3.17}$$

From this point, the reconstruction process develops as described previously. The flow of the processing routine is illustrated in Figure 1.

The breakdown of the global reconstruction into a localized process is made possible by the MR volume-displacement data set. The displacement information provides boundary data for (3.5), enabling a well-posed boundary driven problem to be defined on any arbitrary subzone Ω_z of the global region Ω (Fig. 2). Once a forward solution of (3.5) is available on a subzone, the reconstruction process defined earlier can be applied.

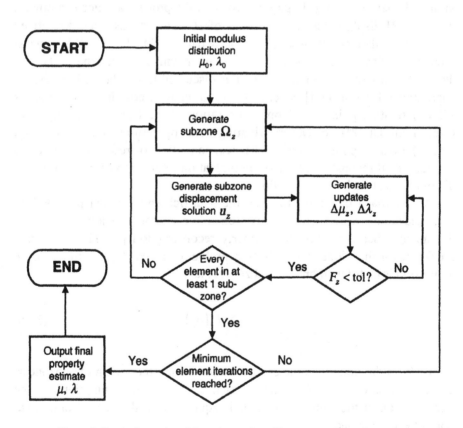

Figure 1. Processing order of the subzone-based image-reconstruction process.

In our approach, the definition of subzones is automated, allowing the reconstruction process to execute in a self-contained fashion whereby globally defined inputs and outputs conceal the subdomain structure of the actual processing. Automation is accomplished by defining overlapping spherical (or, in two dimensions, circular) subzones centered on random seedpoints.

When a spherical subzone does not lie entirely within the global reconstruction domain, the part of the sphere outside Ω is ignored; the resulting subzone has a boundary that is partially inside Ω (therefore spherical), and partially coincident with Γ, the outer surface of the global problem domain. To help maintain smoother boundaries for the randomly generated subzones, element inclusion is determined according to whether the *centroid* of the element lies within radius r of the seed point (i.e., the node that is at the center of the subzone; see Fig. 3). This eliminates the possibility of elements being included within the subzone based only on a single node lying marginally within the specified radius from the subzone center, and so preserves a level of smoothness for the subzone boundary. Once the extent of a subzone is defined by centroid-based element selection, its boundary can be determined automatically and the formulation of the FE forward problem undertaken accordingly.

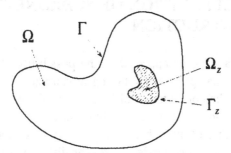

Figure 2. The presence of displacement data throughout global domain Ω having boundary Γ allows the composition of a well-posed boundary problem on subzone domain Ω_z having boundary Γ_z. Figure is after [4].

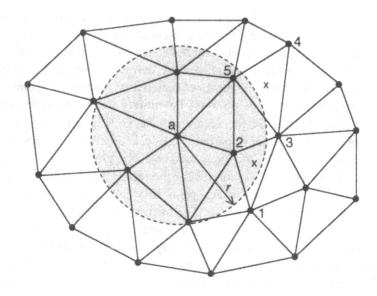

Figure 3. Subzone generation based on element centroids. The subzone in question is centered at node "a" and has radius *r*. Element 123 is included in the subzone because its centroid (marked by "x") is within the radius; element 345 is not included in the subzone because its centroid is outside the radius.

4   PARALLELIZATION OF SUBZONE-BASED RECONSTRUCTION

One advantage of a subzone approach is the possibility of "macroparalleliz-ing" the computational process by taking advantage of subzone independ-ence. By assigning the computation of individual subzone updates to separate processors on a first-come, first-served basis, runtime can be approximately divided by the number of available processors. In macroparallelization, each processor is solely and independently responsible for a particular subzone update; this is in contrast to the usual approach to parallelizing large matrix calculations on multiple processors, which requires significant interprocessor communications. Self-scheduled organization of the subzone calculations allows almost the entire computational load to be divided among the avail-able processors with very little interprocessor overhead.

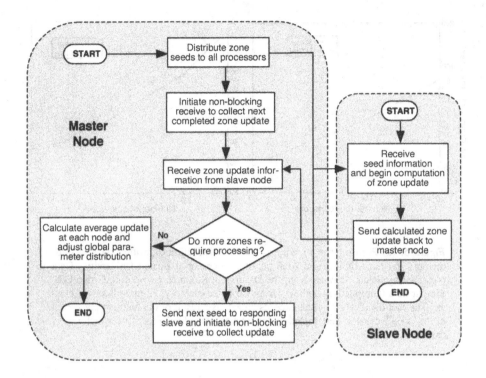

Figure 4. Flowchart of parallelized subzone-based image reconstruction.

We have implemented macroparallelized, subzone-based image reconstruction in Fortran 77 using the message-passing interface (MPI) protocol,
which standardizes communications between processors. After a seed point
is randomly chosen by the "master" processor, subzone generation and parameter updating are handed off to a secondary ("slave") processor. Subzone
results are returned to the master processor and assembled into the global
solution. For large numbers of processors it is better to have one processor
dedicated to overseeing the subzone computations being performed in parallel on the "slave" processors, but with fewer processors one can have the
master processor perform subzone calculations between collecting solutions
from slave processors. A flow chart for this parallelized inversion process is
given in Figure 4.

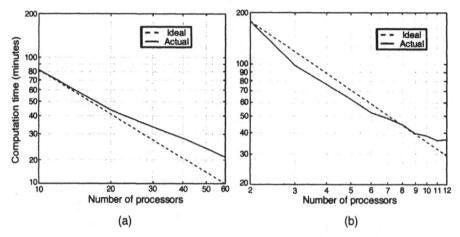

Figure 5. (a) Performance of our parallel reconstruction algorithm on a shared-memory, 64-node SGI Origin 2000 parallel processor at Boston University. (Data compiled by Susan Schwarz from the Dartmouth Research Computing Group.) (b) Similar data (compiled by author) for a distributed-memory, 12-node Beowulf cluster. The fact that "actual" often exceeds "ideal" is a result of the fact that placement of the "ideal" curve is determined by the time assumed for 1 processor, which in this case was too low.

Figure 5a shows the performance (i.e., computation time vs. number of processors used) of our parallel reconstruction algorithm on a shared-memory, 64-node SGI Origin 2000 parallel processor housed at Boston University's Scientific Computing and Visualization Center. Figure 5b shows the algorithm's performance on a distributed-memory Beowulf cluster composed of 12 dual-processing Pentium 4 Xeon nodes located in the Numerical Methods Laboratory at the Thayer School of Engineering, Dartmouth College. With perfect division of labor among processors, runtime should scale as the inverse of the number of processors, entailing a unitary descent with each additional processor on a log-log graph, and this is approximately observed. For these calculations, the master node was used solely for message passing and bookkeeping (no update calculations performed on the master node). For the runs performed on the Beowulf cluster, each node was treated as a single processing node by MPI and loop-level parallelization and multithreading were implemented on the second processor of each node. In both cases, less improvement is obtained for large numbers of nodes or processors. This is to be expected in parallel calculation, but more deterministic (intelligent) zone generation is expected to improve performance for large numbers of processors.

5   INFLUENCE OF SUBZONE SIZE ON RECONSTRUCTION ERROR

Figure 6 shows a simulated phantom geometry for investigation of possible inaccuracies in the assumption of 2D planar conditions in the harmonic displacement field of a symmetric geometry. A spherical inclusion in the center of a rectangular block is simulated. The plane of symmetry indicated in the figure would exhibit 2D plane-strain conditions under static loading, but the viability of 2D planar conditions under harmonic motion cannot be assumed.

Figure 7 shows the Young's-modulus reconstruction results for the simulated phantom in Figure 6 from a subzone-based 2D reconstruction algorithm using the in-plane displacement fields generated from a fully three-dimensional forward calculation. Figure 7a shows the forward-problem material property distribution in the transverse plane in Figure 6; Figure 7b shows the reconstruction results based on a 2D plan-stress assumption; and Figure 7c shows the reconstruction results based on a plane-strain approximation. While some kind of central inclusion is visible in both reconstructions, the overall quality is clearly unsatisfactory for a practical imaging modality.

Figure 8 demonstrates the ability of a three-dimensional, full-volume reconstruction method to account for three-dimensional motion fields in the estimation process and also indicates that subzone size plays a role in determining the quality of reconstructed solutions. Figure 8b shows the results of a global reconstruction based on calculations made with subzones averaging 10 mm in diameter (same simulated phantom as in Figs. 6 and 7, but with the addition of normally-distributed noise truncated to 15% of image range), while Fig. 8c shows the results of a similar calculation initiated under identical starting conditions but with subzones averaging 18 mm in diameter. The diameter of the subzones used for generating Figure 8b was less than the half-wavelength of elastic shear waves in the background medium (i.e., approximately 13 mm); the diameter of the subzones used for generating Figure 8c were greater than this limit. The clear superiority of Figure 8c over Figure 8b suggests that subzone size may have an optimal value, probably based on a tradeoff between error and total runtime (i.e., smaller zones, higher error and shorter runtime; larger zones, lower error and longer runtimes). This optimal value is likely related to the length of the mechanical shear waves in the medium.

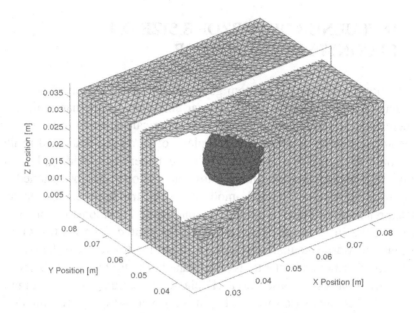

Figure 6. Simulated phantom with homogeneous tetrahedral FE mesh for studying harmonic displacement fields in a symmetric geometry. The block has shear modulus 8.62 kPa and λ modulus 77.58 kPa; the spherical inclusion (here bisected by the imaging plane) is in 3:1 contrast with the block.

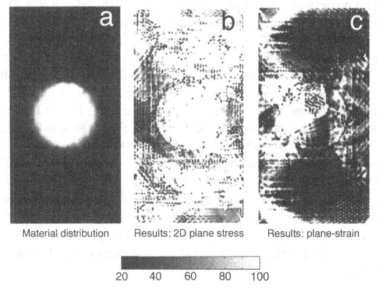

Figure 7. (a) Actual material property distribution in plane shown in Fig. 6. (b, c) Young's-modulus reconstruction results for the simulated phantom in Figure 6. Graybar units are kPa.

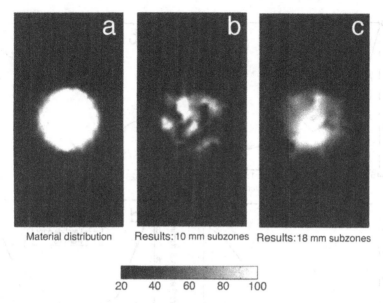

Figure 8. (a) Actual material property distribution in plane shown in Fig. 6. (b, c) In-plane Young's-modulus distributions for 3D subzone-based reconstruction, 10 mm subzones and 18 mm subzones. Graybar units are kPa.

To analyze the dependence of reconstruction error on zone size, we performed a simulation study in which we compared a known forward-problem property distribution to final reconstruction solutions while systematically varying zone radius. We calculated maximum percentage errors for the μ and λ reconstructions and tabulated the computation time for each reconstruction. Figure 9 summarizes the results of this study: the maximum shear modulus error versus zone size (Fig. 9a), the maximum λ error versus zone size (Fig. 9b), runtime versus zone size (Fig. 9c), and all three plots combined on a normalized scale for ease of comparison (Fig. 9d). The length of shear waves within the simulated geometry used for this study was roughly 2.91 cm (i.e., the half wavelength was about 1.455 cm). An optimal zone diameter for this problem, based on an equally weighted cost-function analysis of μ error, λ error, and runtime, is roughly 1.75 cm. An equally weighted cost-function analysis of μ error and λ error only, disregarding runtime, gives the same result, which corresponds roughly to the half wavelength of shear waves in the background medium (i.e., 1.455 cm).

The increase in error found at larger zone sizes in the λ reconstruction may be an effect of greater sensitivity of this parameter to the condition of the Hessian matrix used to generate parameter updates: that is, a larger zone size means a larger Hessian, with consequently poorer conditioning.

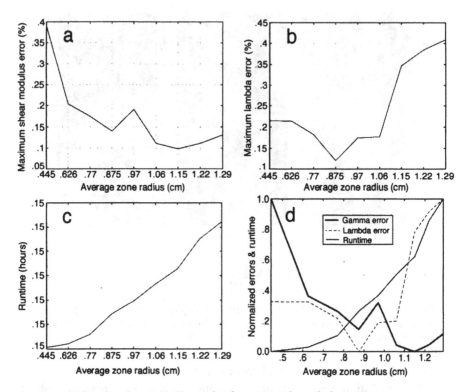

Figure 9. Results of a simulation study of reconstruction solution error vs. zone radius. (a) μ error vs. zone radius. (b) λ error vs. zone radius. (c) Runtime vs. zone radius. (d) All three of the other figures, superimposed.

6   A STATISTICAL APPROACH TO PARAMETER RECONSTRUCTION

A statistical statement of the parameter reconstruction problem can be developed. This provides both an exact definition of the regularization parameter γ (described below), which otherwise must be empirically determined, and calculated variances for each reconstructed parameter θ_k. From a Bayesian perspective [7, 8], one assumes that the parameter set θ is normally distributed with variance τ^2 about a set assumed *a priori*, θ_0 (i.e., $\Theta \sim N(\theta_0, \tau^2 I)$) while the data y are normally distributed about the true distribution $f(\theta)$ with variance σ^2 (i.e., $Y \sim N(f(\theta), \sigma^2 I)$). The probability of a particular parameter set θ, given a specific data set y, is given by

$$p(\theta \mid y) = \frac{p(y,\theta)}{p(y)} = \frac{p(y \mid \theta)p(\theta)}{p(y)} \qquad (3.18)$$

The most probable θ is defined by the solution of

$$\max_{\theta}\{\ln p(\theta \mid y)\} = \max_{\theta}\{\ln p(y \mid \theta) + \ln p(\theta) - \ln p(y)\} \qquad (3.19)$$

For a multivariate, normally distributed system, the probability density functions $p(y \mid \theta, \sigma^2)$ and $p(\theta, \tau^2)$ are given by

$$p(y \mid \theta, \sigma^2) = (2\pi\sigma^2)^{-N_O/2} \exp\left(-\frac{1}{2\sigma^2}\|y - f(\theta)\|^2\right) \qquad (3.20)$$

and $\qquad p(\theta, \tau^2) = (2\pi\tau^2)^{-N_P/2} \exp\left(-\frac{1}{2\tau^2}\|\theta - \theta_0\|^2\right). \qquad (3.21)$

where N_O is the number of observations and N_P is the size of the parameter set being imaged. If σ^2 and τ^2 are known, the constants $\ln(2\pi\sigma^2)^{-N_O/2}$ and $\ln(2\pi\tau^2)^{-N_P/2}$ (which result from the substitution of (3.20) and (3.21) into (3.19)) are irrelevant in the maximization problem. Additionally, $p(y)$ has no dependence on θ and the term $\max_{\theta}\{\ln p(y)\}$ in (3.19) can be ignored. The maximization problem is then written as

$$\theta = \arg\max_{\theta}\left\{-\frac{1}{2\sigma^2}\|y - f(\theta)\|^2 - \frac{1}{2\tau^2}\|\theta - \theta_0\|^2\right\} \qquad (3.22)$$

With a sign change and the substitution $\gamma = \sigma^2/\tau^2$, this yields

$$\theta = \arg\min_{\theta}\left\{\|y - f(\theta)\|^2 + \gamma\|\theta - \theta_0\|^2\right\}, \qquad (3.23)$$

a formulation also known as the *Tikhonov problem* because of the additional *a priori* image regularization term it contains, γ (see Ch. 2, Sec. 4.1).

The Bayesian development presented here provides a definition of the regularization factor γ in terms of the variances of the data measurements and the *a priori* image. Approximations to these variances, $\hat{\sigma}^2$ and $\hat{\tau}^2$, are given by

$$\hat{\sigma}^2 = \frac{1}{N_{PI}} \sum_{API} \frac{1}{N_O - N_P} \|y - f(\theta)\|^2 \qquad (3.24)$$

and

$$\hat{\tau}^2 = \frac{1}{N_{PI} - 1} \sum_{i=1}^{N_{PI}} (\theta_i - \bar{\theta})^2 \qquad (3.25)$$

for an average *a priori* image value $\bar{\theta}$. In (3.24) and (3.25), *API* stands for "all previous images" from which $\bar{\theta}$ was generated and N_{PI} stands for "number of previous images." The history of reconstructed images can thus be utilized to make ensuing images more accurate and to improve convergence. An iterative Gauss-Newton method is used for solution of the optimization problem in (3.23), producing a variant of (2.19) (remembering that $[\partial f / \partial \theta]$ is the Jacobian matrix [J]):

$$\{\theta_{v+1}\} = \{\theta_v\} + \delta_v \left[\left[\frac{\partial f}{\partial \theta}\right]^{\mathrm{T}} \left[\frac{\partial f}{\partial \theta}\right] + \gamma \mathrm{I} \right]^{-1} \left[\left[\frac{\partial f}{\partial \theta}\right]^{\mathrm{T}} \{y - f(\theta)\} - \gamma(\theta - \theta_0) \right] \qquad (3.26)$$

Evaluating the statistical accuracy of the reconstructed parameter set θ, the covariance matrix $[\mathrm{cov}\{\theta\}]$ is given by

$$\left[\mathrm{cov}\{\theta\}\right] = \sigma^2 \left[\frac{\partial \theta}{\partial y}\right] \left[\frac{\partial \theta}{\partial y}\right]^{\mathrm{T}} \qquad (3.27)$$

The matrix $[\partial \theta / \partial y]$ in (3.27) is found by differentiating (3.26) with respect to y with θ_v held constant:

$$\left[\frac{\partial \theta}{\partial y}\right] = \delta_v \left[\left\{\frac{\partial f}{\partial \theta}\right\}^{\mathrm{T}} \left\{\frac{\partial f}{\partial \theta}\right\} + \gamma \mathrm{I} \right]^{-1} \left[\frac{\partial f}{\partial \theta} \right]^{\mathrm{T}} \qquad (3.28)$$

The variance of a particular parameter value θ_k is given by the diagonal term $[\mathrm{cov}\{\theta\}]_{k,k}$. Computing this variance allows calculation of the confidence interval surrounding a reconstructed parameter value for different accuracies. For example, a 95% confidence interval for the kth parameter estimate can be generated from the covariance matrix by $CI_{95\%}(k) = 1.96 \sqrt{[\mathrm{cov}\{\theta\}]_{k,k}}$.

6   CONCLUSION

MRE remains an imaging technique undergoing rapid development, with considerable understanding and theory left to be discovered. Current research on the subzone reconstruction method seeks to improve the efficiency of the zone decomposition methods and to implement more efficient parallelization techniques. Other work is proceeding to adopt statistically based parameter-lumping algorithms to reduce the overall number of degrees of freedom in the reconstruction problem. MRE techniques in general are also being refined to pursue complex mechanical behaviors in living tissue by including such effects as viscoelasticity, anisotropy, and nonlinearity in their underlying models. This should not only improve the ability of these techniques to accurately image elastic properties in living tissue, but may also provide access to hitherto unexploited contrast mechanisms that could be of significant clinical benefit. Clinical MRE results reported by a variety of research teams continue to indicate that this imaging modality does have the potential to play an important role in the detection and diagnosis of disease.

REFERENCES

[1]   R. Muthupillai et al., "Magnetic resonance elastography by direct visualization of propagating acoustic strain waves." *Science*, Vol. 269, 1995, pp. 1854–1857.

[2]   R. Sinkus et al., "High-resolution tensor MR elastography for breast tumor detection." *Phys. Med. Biol.*, Vol. 45, 2000, pp. 1649–1664.

[3]   D. B. Plewes et al., "Visualization and quantification of breast cancer biomechanical properties with magnetic resonance elastography." *Phys. Med. Biol.*, Vol. 45, 2000, pp. 1591–1610.

[4]   E. E. W. Van Houten et al., "An overlapping subzone technique for MR based elastic property reconstruction." *Magnetic Resonance in Medicine*, Vol. 42, 1999, pp. 779–786.

[5]   D. D. Steele et al., "Three-dimensional static displacement, stimulated echo NMR elasticity imaging." *Phys. Med. Biol.*, Vol. 45, 2000, pp. 1633–1648.

[6]   P. C. Chou and N. J. Pagano, *Elasticity: Tensor, Dyadic, and Engineering Approaches* (New York: Dover Publications, 1967).

[7]   J. Besag, "Digital image processing: Towards Bayesian image analysis." *J. Appl. Statistics*, Vol. 16, 1989, pp. 395–407.

[8]   S. S. Saquib, C. A. Bouman, and K. Sauer, "ML parameter estimation for Markov random fields with applications to Bayesian tomography." *IEEE Trans. Imag. Proc.*, Vol. 7, 1998, pp. 1029–1044.

Chapter 4

MAGNETIC RESONANCE ELASTOGRAPHY: EXPERIMENTAL VALIDATION AND PERFORMANCE OPTIMIZATION

Marvin Doyley, Ph.D. and John Weaver, Ph.D.

1   INTRODUCTION

Malignant tumors, such as scirrhous carcinomas of the breast, are noticeably stiffer and less mobile than surrounding, healthy tissues [1]. These properties form the basis of manual palpation, the standard technique currently employed for the subjective clinical assessment of tissue elasticity for breast-cancer detection.

Despite the recognized success of manual palpation in breast cancer detection [2], there are several inherent limitations associated with this technique that diminish its efficacy. For instance, the vast majority of tumors detected using manual palpation are large (> 1 cm in diameter), late-stage, metastatic, and treatable only by employing the most aggressive therapies [3]. Many tumors can elude detection by manual palpation by virtue of their small size and location within the breast.

Although the shear moduli of malignant tissues are generally several orders of magnitude higher than that of normal tissue [4, 5], none of the traditional medical imaging modalities (magnetic resonance imaging [MRI], diagnostic ultrasound, or x-ray computed tomography) are capable of exploiting the large elasticity contrast that exists between healthy and abnormal tissues. For example, many tumors of the prostate or the breast are barely visible on standard ultrasound examination, despite being much harder than the surrounding tissue. Diffuse diseases such as cirrhosis of the liver are known to stiffen the liver appreciably, yet cirrhotic livers frequently appear normal on conventional ultrasound examination.

These observations are not surprising, because the interactions with tissue that form the bases of these techniques are not correlated with tissue elasticity as such. Nonetheless, several conventional medical imaging modalities can provide information on externally induced internal tissue motion, and from this information various mechanical parameters can be inferred [6]. During the last decade, there has been substantial interest in developing a new medical imaging modality, elastography, for visualizing the mechanical properties of soft tissues. At the core of this technique is the estimation of externally induced internal tissue motion using a conventional medical imaging modality. Although the term "elastography" was originally coined by Ophir et al. [7] to describe their ultrasonic elasticity-imaging approach, the use of ultrasound is not essential. Consequently, several groups, including ours at Dartmouth, have been actively developing elastography based on MRI. Although the field of magnetic resonance elastography (MRE) is immature compared to ultrasound elastography, it is likely that technological advances in MRE will enable it to surpass ultrasound elastography relatively soon. MRI has several features that make it ideally suited for elastographic imaging. For example, all three spatial components of the induced internal tissue displacements can be measured with high precision using magnetic resonance imaging, whereas with ultrasound only the displacement component in the direction of the propagating beam can accurately be measured. This problem is attributable to the anisotropic resolution of current diagnostic ultrasound scanners (i.e., axial resolution is superior to lateral and azimuthal resolution). Furthermore, the sensitivity of MRI is superior to that of ultrasound, which makes it appealing when measuring small (micron-scale) internal tissue displacements.

Elastograms (i.e., shear-modulus images) are typically produced using the three-step process illustrated in Figure 1. The first step in the elastographic image-formation process involves inducing displacements within the tissue by employing an external mechanical stimulus. The spatial distribution of the internal displacement field is dependent not only on the mechanical properties of the underlying tissue structures, but also on external and internal boundary conditions and on the nature of the mechanical stimulation (i.e., quasistatic or harmonic). The second step is to measure the induced internal tissue displacement field by employing an appropriate conventional medical imaging modality such as MRI or diagnostic ultrasound. In the third step, the shear-modulus distribution within the tissue is estimated from the measured displacements by applying a model-based inverse reconstruction technique.

The first two stages of this process will be discussed in this chapter in the context of the prototype clinical MRE imaging system developed at the Dartmouth-Hitchcock Medical Center. We will also report the results of preliminary experiments conducted on phantoms and patients to evaluate and optimize the performance of the prototype system.

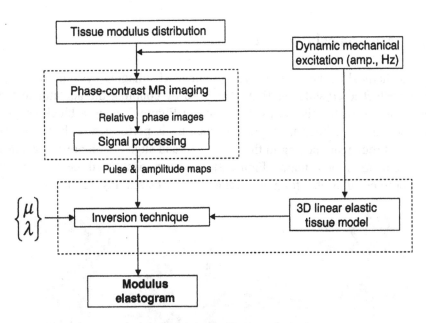

Figure 1. Flow chart of elastographic image formation process.

2   CLINICAL PROTOTYPE MRE IMAGING SYSTEM

A critical step in the elastographic image formation process is the excitation of the tissue under investigation by a mechanical source, either quasistatic or harmonic, coupled to its surface. There is presently no consensus within the imaging research community on whether quasistatic or harmonic excitation is the better approach; the development of MRE has been pursued using both modes of excitation [7–11]. The harmonic approach may have an advantage over the quasistatic method in terms of its ability to accurately recover absolute values of shear modulus. Harmonic waves can also be used to probe tissues that are not readily compressed (e.g., the brain).

A prototype clinical MRE system is currently under development at the Dartmouth-Hitchcock Medical Center to further evaluate the potential of steady-state harmonic elastography. The following section describes the key components of this system, namely, mechanical excitation and displacement estimation.

2.1   Mechanical Excitation

The mechanical actuators employed in our MRE imaging system are based on piezoelectric crystals. Motion is induced by coupling the actuator to the lower surface of the tissue, as illustrated in Figure 2 using a block-shaped phantom. In the clinic, elastographic imaging is performed with the breast pendant through an opening in the breast coil and slightly compressed against the base plate of the actuator (Figure 3). We have constructed the mechanical actuator to be adjustable for a wide range of breast sizes (Figure 4).

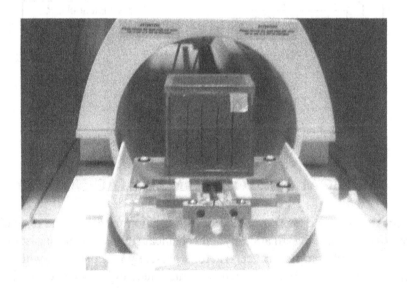

Figure 2. An elasticity phantom, piezoelectric actuator, and head coil. In clinical use, the patient's breast is pendant through the opening of a specialized breast coil and rests on the actuator plate (see Figures 3 and 4).

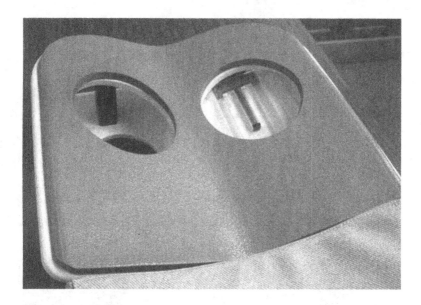

Figure 3. Clinical MRE imaging apparatus with breast coil and mechanical actuator (on right-hand side).

The breast is perturbed mechanically by driving the piezoelectric actuator at a fixed frequency (typically < 300 Hz) using a 150 V peak-to-peak sinusoidal voltage generated by an HP 33120A signal generator. The signal generator is in phase lock with the 10 MHz MRE system clock and feeds its signal to the actuator via a power amplifier (APC Products LE 200/150). Although the displacement on the surface of the tissue is typically on the order of 40 μm, larger displacements are induced inside the breast during steady-state motion by constructive interference of wave fronts propagating in multiple directions.

2.2   Displacement Imaging

Several MRI displacement estimation schemes have been proposed for measuring tissue motion. These techniques include spatial magnetization tagging [8], simulated echo imaging, and phase-contrast imaging [11, 13, 14]. This discussion will focus on the phase-contrast imaging method, since this displacement estimation approach has been incorporated into Dartmouth's prototype clinical MRE imaging system.

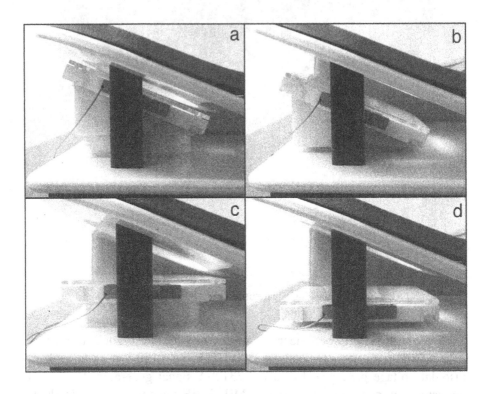

Figure 4. Clinical MRE imaging apparatus. The mechanical actuator is shown at four progressively lower settings (*a* through *d*) in a specialized high-resolution breast coil. The black bar in the foreground is the supporting post of the breast coil.

The premise of phase-contrast MRI is that phase changes will arise when the motion of excited protons occurs in the presence of a magnetic field gradient [13]. The net phase change, $\phi(t)$, incurred over time t from 0 to T when a spin with position vector $\mathbf{r}(t)$ is in the presence of gradient $\mathbf{G}(t)$ is given by

$$\phi = \gamma \int_0^T \mathbf{G}(t) \cdot \mathbf{r}(t)\, dt \qquad (4.1)$$

where γ is the gyromagnetic ratio for the spin. This relates the spin's resonance frequency, ω, to the strength of the local magnetic field, B_0, by $\omega = \gamma B_0$. For a uniform velocity $v(t)$, the position of excited spins is given by

$$\mathbf{r}(t) = \mathbf{r}_0 + \mathbf{v}(t) \tag{4.2}$$

where $\mathbf{r}_0$ is the location of the spin at $t = 0$. Substituting (4.2) into (4.1) gives

$$\phi = \gamma \int_0^T \mathbf{G}(t) \cdot \mathbf{r}_0 \; dt + \int_0^T \mathbf{G}(t) \cdot \mathbf{v}(t) \; dt \tag{4.3}$$

It is interesting to note that phase accumulation will occur due to the presence of both stationary and moving spins. In general, the phase changes due to the stationary spins are used for normal MR images; however, in elastographic imaging only the phase accumulation that occurs due to the motion of moving spins is of interest. Consequently, the phase accumulation associated with stationary spins is eliminated by acquiring the MR signal in phase-cycling mode (i.e., the net phase is computed from the average of two acquisitions that are obtained with opposite motion-encoding gradients). For the situation where spins are undergoing simple harmonic motion, the displacement of spins at equilibrium position $\mathbf{r}_0$ is given by

$$\xi(\mathbf{r},\theta) = \mathbf{r}_0 + \xi_0 \cos\left(k_r \mathbf{r} - \omega t + \theta\right) \tag{4.4}$$

where ξ_0 and ω are the amplitude and angular frequency of vibration, respectively; k_r is the wave number (i.e., $2\pi/\lambda$, where λ is the wavelength); and θ is the initial phase offset between the motion-encoding MR gradient and the mechanical excitation. Muthupillai et al. [13] were the first to demonstrate that a phase accumulation can be generated through the MR field of view (FOV) by applying an oscillating gradient (i.e., $\mathbf{G}(t) = \mathbf{G}_0 \cos(\theta - \omega t)$) to the tissue for a duration T. The phase accumulation resulting from a particle undergoing simple harmonic motion is given by

$$\phi(\mathbf{r},\theta) = \gamma \int_0^T \mathbf{G}_0 \cdot \xi_0 \cos\left(k_r \mathbf{r} - \omega t + \theta\right) dt$$

$$= \frac{2\gamma NT(\mathbf{G}_0 \cdot \xi_0)}{\pi} \sin\left(k_r \mathbf{r}\right) \tag{4.5}$$

Here, N is the number of gradient cycles in the interval T. Snapshots of the propagating wavefront are obtained as function of time by varying the initial phase offset between the motion encoding gradient and mechanical actuator. (The signal generator that drives the mechanical actuator is phase-locked with the MR system clock.)

Figure 5 shows the pulse sequence and the synchronized motion. The phase-contrast method generates the amplitude and relative phase of motion at each point in the image by fitting the phase of the measured image at each position to a sinusoidal function of the relative phase, θ, between the motion encoding gradient and the piezoelectric actuators inducing motion. Spurious phases are removed by cycling the sign of the motion encoding gradient and subtracting the phase of the signal at each position, thus removing spurious phases.

Figure 6 shows examples of amplitude and phase of the propagating wave obtained using the pulse sequence shown in Figure 5. It is important to note that the amplitude and phase are computed by performing a fast Fourier transform for each pixel over a number of phase offsets (typically four to eight) between the applied motion and the encoding gradients. Although these measurement were made under steady-state conditions, the development of wavelike behavior is discernable in both the phase and amplitude images. However, the wave propagation mechanics are fairly complex even for this simple case, due to asymmetric boundary conditions.

Only one displacement component can be measured at a given time using phase-contrast MR imaging. Consequently, the three-dimensional displacement vector at each pixel location is reconstructed from three independent acquisitions.

4   PERFORMANCE ASSESSMENT

4.1   Detectability of Low-Contrast Lesions

A key requirement of any diagnostic imaging system is the ability to detect low-contrast focal lesions. Therefore, it is desirable that our imaging system, in addition to having low-contrast detectability, be able to characterize focal lesions. This could potentially be used as the basis for differentiating between different tumor types.

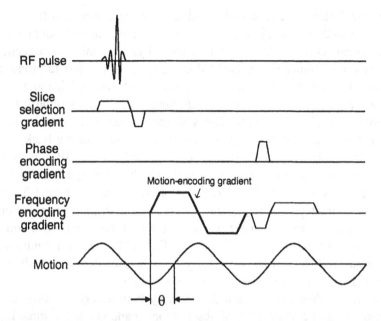

RF pulse

Slice
selection
gradient

Phase
encoding
gradient

Motion-encoding gradient

Frequency
encoding
gradient

Motion

θ

Figure 5. A gradient-echo-based, phase-contrast, motion-imaging pulse sequence for detecting the steady-state harmonic motion within the imaging volume. An offline signal generator coupled to the motion-encoding gradient frequency by trigger pulses on the RF channel is used to drive the piezocrystal actuators at phase offset θ from the motion-encoding gradients. By varying θ and recording the resulting output signal from the sequences, the motion field within the imaging volume can be reconstructed.

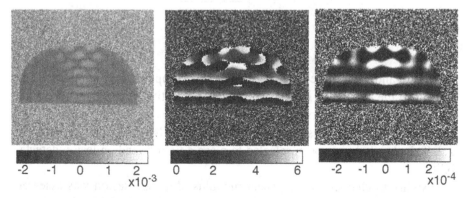

-2 -1 0 1 2
          $\times 10^{-3}$

0 2 4 6

-2 -1 0 1 2
          $\times 10^{-4}$

Figure 6. MR images obtained from the central plane of a homogeneous elastographic imaging phantom using the phase-contrast imaging sequence shown in Fig. 5. Left, the amplitude in the x direction; center, the phase distribution corresponding to the image shown at left; right, displacement image computed from the amplitude and phase images.

Figure 7 shows examples of simulated spherical tumors with sizes ranging from 5 to 20 mm in diameter. They were manufactured from porcine skin
gelatin, formaldehyde, distilled water, and ethylenediamine tetra-acetic acid.
Each simulated tumor was embedded in a soft gelatin matrix to produce contrast-detail phantoms containing single lesions of varying size and modulus
contrast. Figure 8 shows a set of MR magnitude images obtained from a
contrast-detail phantom containing a simulated tumor 10 mm in diameter.
The modulus contrast between the simulated tumor and the background is
high (9:1) in this case. The inclusion is discernible in the MR magnitude image due to the presence of copper sulfate (which is acting as an MR contrast
agent). Figures 9 and 10 show examples of elastograms obtained from high-
and low-contrast phantoms, respectively. Note that all four inclusions are
discernible in the high-contrast phantom, but that the 5 mm inclusion in the
low-contrast phantom is not visualized. Figure 11 shows a contrast-detail
curve measured by performing an objective contrast-detail analysis on elastograms similar to those shown in Figures 9 and 10.

Figure 11 shows that lesion detectability is inversely proportional to lesion size. This is consistent with observations made in conventional imaging
modalities [15]. Further, although all lesions can be detected, it is not possible to accurately characterize the elastic moduli of very small inclusions. The
general premise of contrast-detail analysis is that the likelihood of detecting a
lesion can be expressed in the form of contrast-to-noise ratio (CNR), which is
defined in elastography as [16, 17]

$$\text{CNR} = \sqrt{\frac{2\left(\hat{\mu}_L - \hat{\mu}_B\right)^2}{\sigma_L^2 + \sigma_B^2}} \tag{4.6}$$

where $\hat{\mu}_L$ and $\hat{\mu}_B$ are the mean shear modulus computed over similarly sized
regions in the lesion and background tissue, respectively, and σ_L^2 and σ_B^2 are
the variance of shear modulus in the lesion and background tissue, respectively. We consider a lesion detected when the CNR is greater or equal to
2.2. This threshold has been selected to place a tight bound on lesion detectability.

Ability to characterize the shear modulus of a focal lesion was assessed
by comparing the mean shear modulus recovered over the inclusion relative
to independent estimates of shear modulus obtained through mechanical
testing. The reconstructed object is considered accurately characterized if the

mean shear modulus computed in the lesion is within 2% of the independently-estimated value.

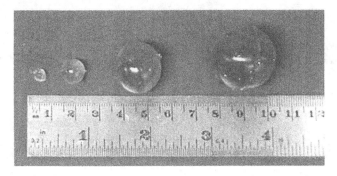

Figure 7. Spherical gelatin inclusions used to simulate focal lesions. In color the inclusions would be green due to the presence of copper sulphate, which is used as a contrast agent to allow the position and extent of the inclusion to be discernible in the MR magnitude images.

5   PRELIMINARY CLINICAL EVALUATION

We have conducted a pilot study on healthy volunteers to gain insight into the performance of our MR data acquisition system in preparation for clinical trials and to compare the shear moduli that we have recovered from normal breast tissues to published breast-elastography data.

Figures 12 and 13 show representative MR magnitude and shear-modulus images obtained from healthy breasts. Figure 12 also shows Poisson's-ratio (MR magnitude) and covariance images. The lower Poisson's-ratio levels within the fatty tissues may be an indication of the lower percentage of water content of these tissues compared to fibroglandular tissues, as Poisson's ratio is related to the compressibility of a material, which is likely reflective of water content. The right-hand panels in Figures 12 and 13 show the corresponding elastograms, calculated using 3D overlapping subzone inversion as described in Ch. 3. The fibroglandular tissue is the dark, central region in the MR magnitude images and the fatty tissue is the light region in the MR magnitude images. Note that the fibroglandular tissues are stiffer (brighter) than the fatty tissues. This is consistent with observations made from independent mechanical testing [5]. Furthermore, there is good correlation between the elastograms and the anatomic features in the MR magnitude images.

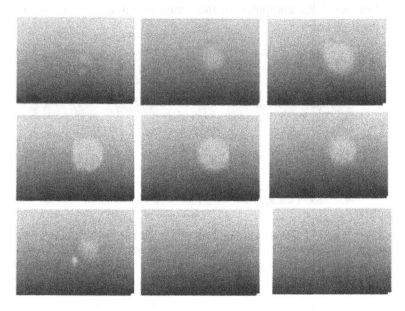

Figure 8. Axial MR magnitude images obtained from a 3.5 cm × 4.1 cm × 16 mm FOV in the center of a phantom containing a 10 mm diameter inclusion. The image planes are spaced 3 mm apart along the 3.5 cm dimension of the phantom; read slices row-wise from top to bottom. The elastic modulus contrast between the simulated tumor and the background is 9:1. An elastogram of the same phantom is shown in Fig. 9b.

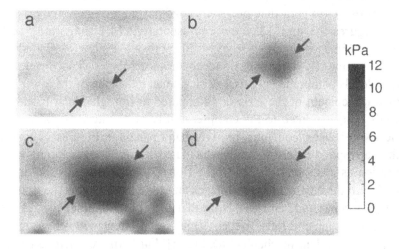

Figure 9. Axial elastogram obtained from the central plane of high-contrast (9:1) elasticity phantoms containing (a) 5 mm, (b) 10 mm, (c) 18 mm, and (d) 25 mm diameter lesions. Each image is approximately 4 × 5 cm.

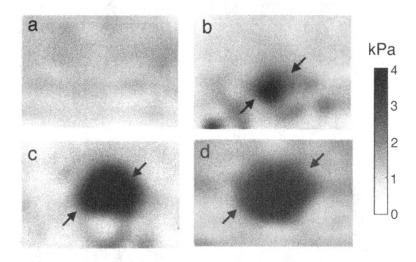

Figure 10. Axial elastograms obtained from the central planes of low-modulus-contrast (2:1) elasticity phantoms containing (a) 5 mm, (b) 10 mm, (c) 18 mm, and (d) 25 mm diameter lesions. Each image is approximately 4 × 5 cm.

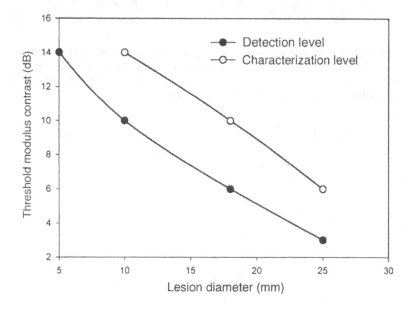

Figure 11. Contrast-detail curve showing the threshold modulus required to detect and characterize focal lesions.

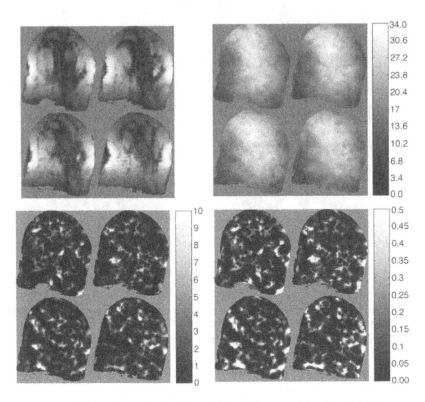

Figure 12. Examples of MR magnitude (top left) and shear-modulus (top right) images obtained from the central plane of a healthy breast. Shear-modulus grayscale units are in units of kPa. Images at lower left are for the magnitude of the covariance; images at lower right are the Poisson's ratios.

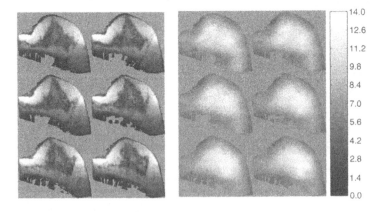

Figure 13. MR magnitude (left) and shear-modulus (right) images obtained from the central plane of a healthy breast. Shear-modulus grayscale units are kPa.

REFERENCES

[1] W. Anderson, *Pathology* (St. Louis, MO: Mosby, 1953).
[2] L. M. Newcomer et al., "Detection method and breast carcinoma histology." *Cancer*, Vol. 95, 2002, pp. 470–477.
[3] L. Keith et al., "Are mammography and palpation sufficient for breast cancer screening? A dissenting opinion." *Journal of Women's Health & Gender-Based Medicine*, Vol. 11(1), 2002, pp. 17–25.
[4] A. P. Savazyn et al., "Elasticity imaging as a new modality of medical imaging for cancer detection." *Premieres Journées D'études*, 1994.
[5] T. A. Krouskop et al., "Elastic moduli of breast and prostate tissues under compression." *Ultrasonic Imaging*, Vol. 20(4), 1998, pp. 260–274.
[6] J. Ophir et al., "Elastography: A systems approach." *International Journal of Imaging Systems and Technology*, Vol. 8, 1997, pp. 89–93.
[7] J. Ophir et al., "Elastography—a quantitative method for imaging the elasticity of biological tissues." *Ultrasonic Imaging*, Vol. 13, 1991, pp. 111–134.
[8] J. B. Fowlkes et al., "Magnetic-resonance imaging techniques for detection of elasticity variation." *Med. Phys.*, Vol. 22(11 Pt 1), 1995, pp. 1771–1778.
[9] D. B. Plewes et al., "Visualizing tissue compliance with MR imaging." *J. Magn. Reson. Imaging*, Vol. 5(6), 1995, 733–738.
[10] R. Muthupillai and R. L. Ehman, "Magnetic resonance elastography." *Nat. Med.*, Vol. 2(5), 1996, pp. 601–603.
[11] R. Sinkus et al., "High-resolution tensor MR elastography for breast tumour detection." *Phys. Med. Biol.*, Vol. 45(6), 2000, pp. 1649–1664.
[12] E. E. Van Houten et al., "Initial in vivo experience with steady-state subzone-based MR elastography of the human breast." *J. Magn. Reson. Imaging*, Vol. 17(1), 2003, pp. 72–78.
[13] R. Muthupillai et al., "Interleaved spiral acquisition for MR elastography." *Radiology*, Vol. 201, 1996, p. 361.
[14] J. B. Weaver et al., "Magnetic resonance elastography using 3D gradient echo measurements of steady-state motion." *Med. Phys.*, Vol. 28(8), 2001, pp. 1620–1628.
[15] B. W. Pogue et al., "Contrast detailed analysis for detection and reconstruction with near-infrared diffuse tomography." *Med. Phys.*, Vol. 27(12), 2000, pp. 2693–2699.
[16] M. Bilgen, "Target detectability in acoustic elastography." *IEEE Trans. Ultrason. Ferroelectr. Freq. Control*, Vol. 6(5), 1997, pp. 1128–1133.
[17] P. Chaturvedi et al., "Testing the limitations of 2-D companding for strain imaging using phantoms." *IEEE Trans. Ultrasonics Ferroelectrics & Frequency Control*, Vol. 45, 1998, pp. 1022–1031.

Chapter 5

ELECTRICAL IMPEDANCE SPECTROSCOPY: THEORY

Hamid Dehghani, Ph.D. and Nirmal K. Soni, M.Tech.

1   INTRODUCTION

In electrical impedance spectroscopy (EIS), electrodes are placed in contact with the surface of the domain being imaged (e.g., head, breast, limb) and voltages or currents are applied. The induced currents and/or voltages are measured at some or all of the electrodes, which allows a map of the internal distribution of conductivity (σ) and permittivity (ε) in the domain of interest to be derived. EIS differs from microwave imaging spectroscopy, which also maps σ and ε, primarily in its lower operating band (≈ 1 kHz to 10 MHz). When tomographic techniques are used to form electrical impedance images from boundary measurements, as in our work, EIS is often referred to as electrical impedance *tomography*.

EIS is of interest because the electrical properties of tissue can vary significantly with physiology and pathology. Of particular importance in breast imaging are the differences between normal tissue and carcinoma (Fig. 1). Not only are these electrical properties distinct in the 10^{-2}–10^2 MHz range, but for conductivity the contrast increases with frequency. Many groups have, therefore, emphasized the importance of obtaining spectral information to help identify tumors [1–3]. Our group at Dartmouth has constructed an EIS system that can be operated at any desired frequency from 10 KHz to 10 MHz. This system is described further in the next chapter.

The task of mapping the electrical property distribution of a tissue volume using measurements of low-frequency surface currents and potentials is a difficult one. First, the electrical-property features of tissue, while attractive candidates for imaging because they offer large intrinsic contrast, are encoded as small, nonlocalized changes in surface currents and potentials. Second, surface measurements are intrinsically less sensitive to changes in electrical properties deep within the tissue being imaged, making EIS's depth resolution relatively poor. Third, the measured electrical response is a non-linear function of the tissue electrical properties, and this nonlinearity, coupled to the spatial dependence of the sensitivity map to property changes, makes for a challenging parameter-estimation problem. (Some groups have experimented with tomographic approaches that linearize the relationship between electrical property change and change in measured response [4].)

All of these difficulties can be overcome with careful design of both algorithms and hardware. Like the other imaging modalities represented in this volume, we have opted for an iterative image-reconstruction approach based on finite element (FE) modeling.

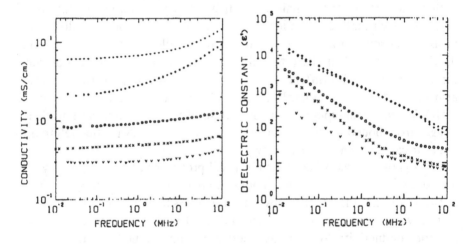

Figure 1. Conductivity and dielectric constant of breast carcinoma as a function of frequency. (∗) = sample from central part of tumor, (+) = sample from tissue surrounding tumor, (o) = sample consisting mainly of fatty tissue containing infiltrating tumor cells, (x) = peripheral sample located relatively far from central part of tumor, and (v) = normal breast tissue. From Surowiec et al. [5].

2   THE PHYSICAL MODEL

2.1   Conditions and Assumptions

EIS requires a numerical model that links surface voltages and currents, both injected and measured, to the electrical-property distribution within the target volume. Such a model can be derived from Maxwell's equations if several simplifying assumptions are invoked. In an inhomogeneous medium, Maxwell's equations can be written as

$$\nabla \times \mathbf{E} = -\frac{\partial \mathbf{B}}{\partial t} \tag{5.1}$$

and
$$\nabla \times \mathbf{H} = \mathbf{J} + \frac{\partial \mathbf{D}}{\partial t} \tag{5.2}$$

where $\mathbf{E}$ is the electric field, $\mathbf{B}$ is the magnetic induction, $\mathbf{H}$ is the magnetic field, $\mathbf{J}$ is the electric current density, and $\mathbf{D}$ is the electric displacement. Assuming a simple linear isotropic medium, it is also true that

$$\mathbf{D} = \varepsilon \mathbf{E}, \ \mathbf{B} = \mu \mathbf{H}, \text{ and } \mathbf{J} = \sigma \mathbf{E} \tag{5.3}$$

where ε is the permittivity, μ is the magnetic permeability, and σ is the conductivity of the medium.

In EIS, further assumptions can be made:

1. *Time harmonic variables.* Assuming that the injected currents and voltages are time-harmonic at a given radian frequency ω and that $\mathbf{J} = \mathbf{J}^o + \mathbf{J}^s$ (where $\mathbf{J}^o$ is the ohmic current, $\mathbf{J}^o = \sigma \mathbf{E}$, and $\mathbf{J}^s$ is the source current), (5.1) and (5.2) can be written

$$\nabla \times \mathbf{E} = -i\omega\mu\mathbf{H} \quad \text{and} \quad \nabla \times \mathbf{H} = (\sigma + i\omega\varepsilon)\mathbf{E} + \mathbf{J}^s \tag{5.4}$$

   where $i = \sqrt{-1}$.

2. *Quasistatic assumption.* The exact expression for $\mathbf{E}$ can be given as

$$\mathbf{E} = -\nabla\Psi - \frac{\partial \mathbf{A}}{\partial t} \tag{5.5}$$

where Ψ is the electric potential and $\mathbf{A}$ is the magnetic vector potential. If magnetic induction of electric fields is neglected—as it can be if the time variation in $\mathbf{A}$ is small relative to the spatial gradient in Ψ—then the static form holds (i.e., $\mathbf{E} = -\nabla\Psi$). A problem in which the static form of (5.5) is used even when (relatively slow) time variation is present is termed *quasistatic*.

3. *Isotropic tissue properties.* Although many tissues are clearly electrically anisotropic, isotropy is assumed in EIS to make the problem tractable. In the breast, this is probably a more reasonable assumption than in some other body tissues (e.g., muscle), although evidence of mechanical anisotropy in the breast does exist [6].

Under these conditions (i.e., quasistatic fields in a linear, isotropic medium), Maxwell's equations can be recast as

$$\mathbf{E} = -\nabla\Psi \tag{5.6}$$

and
$$\nabla \times \mathbf{H} = (\sigma + i\omega\varepsilon)\mathbf{E} + \mathbf{J}^s \tag{5.7}$$

Taking the divergence of both sides of (5.7) and substituting (5.6) into the result, we obtain

$$\nabla \cdot (\sigma + i\omega\varepsilon)\nabla\Psi = 0 \tag{5.8}$$

Here, $\varepsilon = \varepsilon_0\varepsilon_r$, where $\varepsilon_0 = 8.854 \times 10^{-12}$ F/m is the absolute permittivity of free space and ε_r is the (unitless) relative electrical permittivity. The potential, Ψ, is a function of σ and ε, which are themselves functions of position (assuming time invariance). Below, for brevity, we employ the notation $\sigma^* = \sigma + i\omega\varepsilon$, where σ^* is referred to as the "complex-valued conductivity."

2.2 Boundary Conditions

In order to obtain a reasonable model for EIS from the equations above, appropriate boundary conditions must be specified. Several boundary conditions are widely used:

1. *Continuum model.* This model assumes that there are no electrodes and that the injected current or applied voltage is a continuous function of position around the periphery of the imaging domain.

2. *Gap model.* This model assumes that the injected current or the applied voltages are uniform under each electrode, i.e., that for each node under an electrode the current is equal to I_ℓ (total current for that electrode) divided by the area of the electrode, and that for nodes elsewhere on the boundary the current is zero.

3. *Shunt model.* This model takes into account the shunting effect of the electrode, i.e., assumes that the potential under each electrode is constant. This model improves over the gap model, where one assumes that the excitation signal is constant under each electrode, by ensuring that the resultant voltage or current is also constant.

4. *Complete electrode model.* This model takes into account both the shunting effect of the electrode and the impedance between the electrode and tissue at the point of contact. Using this boundary condition, the EIS model in (5.8) is augmented with the following constraints:

$$\Psi + z_\ell \sigma^* \frac{\partial \Psi}{\partial n} = V_\ell, \ x \in e_\ell, \ \ell = 1, 2, \ldots, O_E \qquad (5.9)$$

$$\int_{e_\ell} \sigma^* \frac{\partial \Psi}{\partial n} dS = I_\ell, \ x \in e_\ell, \ \ell = 1, 2, \ldots, O_E \qquad (5.10)$$

$$\sigma^* \frac{\partial \Psi}{\partial n} = 0, \ x \in \partial\Omega \backslash \cup_\ell^{O_E} e_\ell \qquad (5.11)$$

where O_E is the number of electrodes, x is a point in the domain, z_ℓ is the effective contact impedance between the ℓth electrode and the tissue, I_ℓ is the applied current at the ℓth electrode, V_ℓ is the resulting voltage at the ℓth electrode, and e_ℓ denotes the portion of the problem domain occupied by electrode ℓ. The notation "$x \in \partial\Omega \backslash \cup_\ell^{O_E} e_\ell$" indicates a boundary point that is not under any electrode.

3   IMAGE RECONSTRUCTION

3.1   Problem Formulation

Image reconstruction begins with a set of O_{IM} boundary data values, Φ_i, that are measured by electrodes in contact with the surface of an object. Φ can represent either the measured voltage due to injected current or vice versa. Because current and voltage may be measured simultaneously at each electrode, O_{IM} may be greater than O_E.

A general approach to imaging the interior spatial distribution of electrical properties is to minimize the squared difference between these O_{IM} measured values and a set of O_{IM} quantities derived from some numerical model, that is, to minimize the error function

$$\chi^2 = \sum_{i=1}^{O_{IM}} \left(\Phi_i^m - \Phi_i^c \right)^2 \tag{5.12}$$

where m denotes a measured value and c denotes its model-calculated counterpart. The σ^* distribution that minimizes χ^2 provides the desired spatial map or image of the object electrical properties. Finding this distribution requires that we set the derivative of (5.12) with respect to σ^* equal to zero, which, through application of Newton's method to solve the resulting nonlinear system of equations, generates an expression for an update vector, $\Delta\sigma^*$ (in matrix notation):

$$\left\{ \Delta\sigma^* \right\} = \left[J^T J + \lambda I \right]^{-1} \left[J^T \right] \left\{ \Phi^m - \Phi^c \right\} \tag{5.13}$$

Here, $\{\Delta\sigma^*\}$ is a vector of length L (the number of estimated parameter values); $\{\Phi^m - \Phi^c\}$ is a vector of length O_{IM}; λ is a regularization parameter (see Ch. 2, Sec. 4.1); [I] is the $L \times L$ identity matrix; and [J] is the $O_{IM} \times L$ Jacobian matrix $\partial\Phi^c / \partial\sigma^*$, the matrix of derivatives of the O_{IM} calculated measurements Φ_i^c with respect to each of the L estimated parameter values. The Jacobian, which expresses the sensitivity of the measurements to infinitesimal changes in σ^* at each position in the property domain discretization (e.g., node in the property mesh), has the form

$$[\mathbf{J}] = \begin{bmatrix} \dfrac{\partial \Phi_1^c}{\partial \sigma_1^*} & \dfrac{\partial \Phi_1^c}{\partial \sigma_2^*} & \cdots & \dfrac{\partial \Phi_1^c}{\partial \sigma_L^*} \\[2ex] \dfrac{\partial \Phi_2^c}{\partial \sigma_1^*} & \dfrac{\partial \Phi_2^c}{\partial \sigma_2^*} & \cdots & \dfrac{\partial \Phi_2^c}{\partial \sigma_L^*} \\[2ex] \vdots & \vdots & \ddots & \vdots \\[2ex] \dfrac{\partial \Phi_{O_{IM}}^c}{\partial \sigma_1^*} & \dfrac{\partial \Phi_{O_{IM}}^c}{\partial \sigma_2^*} & \cdots & \dfrac{\partial \Phi_{O_{IM}}^c}{\partial \sigma_L^*} \end{bmatrix} \qquad (5.14)$$

$\{\Phi^c\}$ is calculated from the current estimate of $\{\sigma^*\}$ using the techniques for solving the forward problem described in Chapter 2. In the following section, the determination of [J] is described. With these tools in hand, it is possible to solve (5.13) iteratively to find the $\{\sigma^*\}$ that minimizes (5.12) and becomes the resultant image.

3.2 The Jacobian

The Jacobian, also known as the sensitivity or weight matrix, maps a small change in electrical properties to a small change in measured boundary data:

$$\Phi + \Delta\Phi \Leftrightarrow \left[\mathbf{J}\left(\sigma^* + \Delta\sigma^*\right) \right] \qquad (5.15)$$

for a small change Δ. The strict definition of [J] is, therefore, $\partial\Phi/\partial\sigma^*$. There are three common methods of calculating [J], which are outlined below.

1. The perturbation method. The perturbation method invokes finite difference calculus to directly calculate the Jacobian, one pixel at a time. The basis of the method is that given a domain to be imaged, each pixel (e.g., node or element) in turn is altered in conductivity by a change $\Delta\sigma^*$ for each excitation pattern. A resulting change $\Delta\Phi$ is measured (calculated) at each electrode and is used to approximate the corresponding continuum derivative as an entry in the requisite location of the Jacobian matrix. The computation time is proportional to the number of excitation patterns times the number of pixels in the image.

2. *The direct method.* In the direct method, the Jacobian can be calculated by differentiating (5.8) with respect to σ^*. This produces

$$\nabla \cdot \sigma^* \nabla \Phi' + \nabla \cdot \sigma^{*\prime} \nabla \Phi = 0 \tag{5.16}$$

where the prime indicates differentiation with respect to σ^*. Equation (5.16) is an inhomogeneous PDE in $\partial_\sigma \cdot \Phi$ which has the identical form of (5.8) with the addition of a forcing term involving $\sigma^{*\prime}$ and Φ. Since the derivative quantities in the Jacobian are needed at the current estimate of σ^*, the forcing term can be computed everywhere in the domain. Discretization of (5.16) onto a linear algebraic system can be achieved by the same method employed to solve (5.8). In discrete matrix form, the solution to (5.16) can be written as

$$\left\{ \frac{\partial \Phi}{\partial \sigma^*} \right\} = -\left[A \right]^{-1} \left(\left[\frac{\partial A}{\partial \sigma^*} \right] \{\Phi\} \right) \tag{5.17}$$

Here, $[A]^{-1}$ and Φ are already known from the forward solution, which only leaves the calculation of $\partial A/\partial \sigma^*$, which can be determined one pixel (node, element) at a time by

$$\frac{\partial A_{ij}}{\partial \sigma_k^*} = -\left\langle \varphi_k \nabla \varphi_j \cdot \nabla \varphi_i \right\rangle \tag{5.18}$$

where φ is the shape function associated with each node or element i, j, or k (analogous to the basis function described in Ch. 2). In practice, the Jacobian is assembled on a column-by-column basis. The computation time is proportional to the number of excitation patterns times the number of reconstruction parameter nodes.

3. *The adjoint method.* The calculation of the Jacobian by the adjoint method is similar to that described for the near infrared tomography case and is given in [7] as

$$\frac{\partial \Phi}{\partial \sigma^*} = -\int_\Omega \nabla \Phi_D \cdot \nabla \Phi_A \tag{5.19}$$

where Ω is the image domain, Φ_D is the direct forward solution calculated for each excitation pattern, and Φ_A is the adjoint field calculated for each measurement electrode (see Ch. 2).

In our case, the adjoint field is computed by assuming that a current or voltage of unity is injected into the measurement electrode while a current or voltage scaled by $1/(N-1)$ is induced at the $(N-1)$ other electrodes. Here, each row of the Jacobian can be calculated at once using (5.19). The computation time for the entire Jacobian is proportional to the number of excitation patterns times the number of electrodes (adjoint fields), which is significantly less than for the other two methods described above.

4   TRIGONONOMETRIC DRIVING PATTERNS

In EIS it is possible to drive and measure current and voltage at the same electrode simultaneously. This makes possible a wide variety of drive/measure permutations. Since current must flow into the body through at least one electrode and out of the body through at least one other, the minimum excitation pattern is a pair. One paired driving approach is the adjacent method, in which current is injected at two adjacent electrodes (by specifying either the voltage or the current) and potentials are measured at all other sites. A set of measurements can be constructed by exciting more than one pair in turn. This method probes near-surface structure most effectively. Alternatively, current can be passed between two electrodes on opposite sides of the body, and potentials measured at all of the other positions. This configuration probes deeper structure most effectively [8].

A third approach varies the current magnitude across a number of current-injecting electrodes. One class of driving patterns, the trigonometric excitation patterns, was shown by Isaacson [9] to provide maximum sensitivity to structural heterogeneity for a cylindrically symmetric geometry. In this technique, all possible sine and cosine modulations (i.e., those having an integral number of periods) are applied in sequence to the electrodes positioned around the perimeter. That is, for O_E electrodes, O_E-1 passes are made, during which the signal amplitude A_θ for the electrode at angle θ (as measured from the center of the target) is given, on the K th pass, by

$$A_\theta = A \begin{cases} \cos(K\theta) & K = 1,2,\ldots,O_E/2 \\ \sin\big([K-O_E/2]\theta\big) & K = O_E/2+1,\ldots,O_E-1 \end{cases} \tag{5.20}$$

where A is the maximum signal amplitude. In effect, the high spatial frequencies (higher-K passes) maximize the distinguishability of near-surface structure while low spatial frequencies (lower-K passes) maximize the distinguishability of deep structure.

As noted above, the contact impedance at each electrode (generally in the range of a few tens of ohms) causes an unknown voltage drop to occur at each electrode that passes current. When trigonometric excitation patterns are applied, all electrodes pass current simultaneously and suffer from an unknown voltage drop. As a countermeasure, we have experimented with an excitation method termed the *synthesized trigonometric pattern*, which works as follows.

If the system comprising the target, electrodes, and system electronics is linear with regard to the driving signals, the principle of superposition can be applied. That is, a weighted sum of the voltages and currents from a number of excitation patterns applied sequentially should equal the voltages and currents that would result if all of those excitation patterns were applied simultaneously. Hence, a trigonometric excitation pattern can be synthesized as a weighted sum of a set of currents applied sequentially between each electrode and a fixed reference electrode (Fig. 2) [10]. Since one electrode must be devoted to the role of reference, $O_E - 1$ sub-patterns are summed for each trigonometric excitation pattern where there are O_E electrodes.

Simulation and practice have shown that synthesized trigonometric excitation is, as expected, less susceptible to the effects of electrode contact resistance. However, since noise is compounded during the synthesis process, it is more sensitive to noise. Whether or not it is beneficial to employ, therefore, depends on whether image quality in a given system is degraded more by signal noise or by contact resistance.

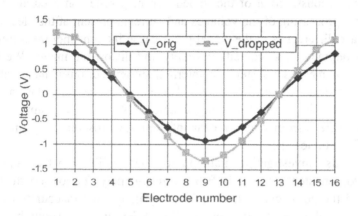

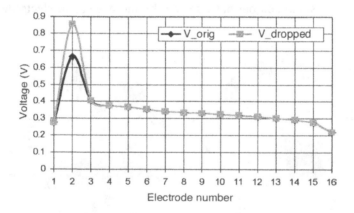

Figure 2. Top: Trigonometric excitation pattern for a 16-electrode system with $K = 1$. "V_orig" is the applied voltage and "V_dropped" is the applied voltage plus simulated contact-impedance drop. Sixteen random contact impedances between $30 \, \Omega$ and $40 \, \Omega$ were assigned to the 16 electrodes. *Bottom*: Same variables for one of the 15 excitation patterns used in synthesizing the trigonometric pattern above. Since for each sub-pattern only one electrode (not counting the reference, not shown) passes current, only one electrode suffers from an unknown voltage drop.

5   DATA CALIBRATION

Quantitative reconstruction of the impedance map relies on accurate measurement and processing of the voltages and currents present at the electrodes, but hardware differences in the signal paths cause interchannel measurement errors that degrade data acquisition quality and distort the image. We have therefore implemented a system for internal, automated, on-demand calibration of the hardware in our EIS system. This hardware instrumentation is described more fully in the following chapter. (Note that our approach to calibration differs from that for near-infrared spectroscopic imaging, discussed in Ch. 10, Sec. 4.)

We are also investigating mathematical data-calibration techniques to combat two persistent artifacts in EIS images, namely, the low-conductivity halo around the periphery of the conductivity image and inaccurate estimation of the global conductivity average (Fig. 3). Experiments show that these artifacts can be smoothed but not removed by more accurate electrode modeling [7].

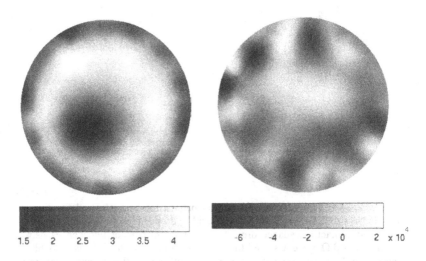

Figure 3. Conductivity (left) and relative permittivity (right) images of an agar phantom with an air core, made using a 16-electrode EIS system operating at 125 kHz. A point-electrode model was used (i.e., one boundary node per electrode). Units of conductivity image are S/m; relative permittivity is unitless. Agar phantom is 10 cm in diameter and 4 cm tall. Air hole is 2 cm in diameter and 2 cm from the edge of the cylinder. The actual conductivity and relative permittivity of the phantom are approximately 2 S/m and 78, respectively. The peripheral ring in the conductivity image and the overall elevation in the conductivity values are artifacts that occur despite the correct identification of the location of the air hole.

We have, therefore, developed a data calibration scheme (so far applied to phantoms only) that corrects data collected from inhomogeneous targets using data from homogeneous simulations and phantoms. This scheme consists of three steps [11]:

1. *Scaling factor determination.* Consider the matrix of boundary current values that is obtained by simulating the imaging of a homogeneous target by an O_E-electrode system applying O_E-1 trigonometric excitation patterns (directly, not using the synthetic scheme noted above). Let $[I_{hs}]$ be the $O_E \times (O_E-1)$ matrix of resulting complex-valued current measurements (where *hs* stands for "homogeneous simulation"). Further, let $[I_{he}]$ be the matrix of currents measured using a homogeneous phantom (where *he* stands for "homogeneous experiment"). A matrix of scaling factors, [SF], also $O_E \times (O_E-1)$, can be calculated by element-by-element division of $[I_{hs}]$ by $[I_{he}]$:

$$SF_{ji} = \frac{(I_{hs})_{ji}}{(I_{he})_{ji}} \qquad (5.21)$$

where (j,i) denotes the jth electrode recording of the ith parameter. When $(I_{he})_{ji} = 0$, SF_{ji} is calculated as an average of adjacent electrode values:

$$SF_{ji} = \frac{SF_{(j-1)i} + SF_{(j+1)i}}{2} \qquad (5.22)$$

Furthermore, these scaling factors are averaged across the electrodes for each excitation pattern to produce a vector of averaged scaling factors, {ASF}, of length O_E-1, where

$$ASF_i = \frac{1}{O_E} \sum_{j=1}^{O_E} SF_{ji}, \quad i = 1,2,...O_E-1 \qquad (5.23)$$

A matrix of experimental measurements from an inhomogeneous target, $[I_{ae}]$ (*ae* stands for "anomaly experiment"), are mapped to a matrix of "anomaly experiment equivalent" (*aee*) values or of "homogeneous experiment equivalent" (*hee*) values through multiplication by the ASF values:

$$(I_{aee})_{ji} = (I_{ae})_{ji} ASF_i \quad \text{and} \quad (I_{hee})_{ji} = (I_{he})_{ji} ASF_i \qquad (5.24)$$

2. *Global property value estimation.* Global target property values are determined by a single-pixel or global average reconstruction that applies the assumption of homogeneity to the scaled data from Step 1. The scaled currents in (5.24), along with the known voltage excitation, are used in a single-pixel forward solution that produces property estimates for both the homogeneous agar phantom (σ_{hg} and $\varepsilon_{r_{hg}}$, where *hg* stands for "homogeneous global") and for the agar phantom with the inclusion or anomaly (σ_{ag} and $\varepsilon_{r_{ag}}$, where *ag* stands for "anomalous global"). These values are used in Step 3.

3. *Offset removal.* The scaled currents from Step 1 for the homogeneous and anomalous cases should, respectively, match forward solutions obtained with (σ_{hg}, $\varepsilon_{r_{hg}}$) and (σ_{ag}, $\varepsilon_{r_{ag}}$) as initial estimates. Due to various experimental errors (contact impedances, hardware drift, etc.), this is not true. Therefore, we calculate an offset between the modeled currents (i.e., forward-solution currents based on global property values from Step 2) and the scaled measured currents (the final product of the calibration process). This offset is calculated both for the homogeneous phantom and the phantom with an anomaly. We denote the offset between measured and modeled currents for a homogeneous phantom (with the modeled currents based on σ_{hg} and $\varepsilon_{r_{hg}}$) as I_{oh} (where *oh* stands for "offset, homogeneous"); and we denote the offset between measured and modeled currents for the anomalous phantom (with the modeled currents based on σ_{ag} and $\varepsilon_{r_{ag}}$) as I_{oa} (where *oa* stands for "offset, anomalous"). The calibrated currents are then given by

$$I_{ac} = I_{acc} - \left(I_{he} - I_{hs}\right) - \left(I_{oa} - I_{oh}\right) \qquad (5.25)$$

Here, I_{ac} (where *ac* stands for "anomalous, calibrated") is used along with the global property values σ_{ag} and $\varepsilon_{r_{ag}}$ as the data input for final image reconstruction.

A flow chart of the calibration scheme is given in Figure 4 and an example of its effect is shown in Figure 5. The peripheral low-conductivity artifact has been removed and the global conductivity value is much closer to that of the agar phantom (approximately 2 S/m). Transfer of this technique to clinical breast imaging will require the construction of appropriate calibration phantoms for the breast.

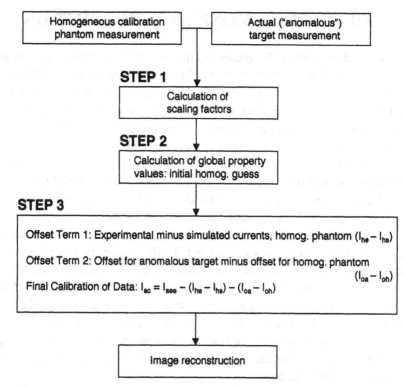

```
┌─────────────────────────────┐   ┌─────────────────────────────┐
│  Homogeneous calibration    │   │  Actual ("anomalous")       │
│  phantom measurement        │   │  target measurement         │
└─────────────────────────────┘   └─────────────────────────────┘
```

STEP 1

```
┌─────────────────────────────┐
│  Calculation of             │
│  scaling factors            │
└─────────────────────────────┘
```

STEP 2

```
┌─────────────────────────────┐
│  Calculation of global property │
│  values: initial homog. guess   │
└─────────────────────────────┘
```

STEP 3

Offset Term 1: Experimental minus simulated currents, homog. phantom ($I_{he} - I_{hs}$)

Offset Term 2: Offset for anomalous target minus offset for homog. phantom

$$(I_{oa} - I_{oh})$$

Final Calibration of Data: $I_{ac} = I_{aee} - (I_{he} - I_{hs}) - (I_{oa} - I_{oh})$

```
┌─────────────────────────────┐
│  Image reconstruction       │
└─────────────────────────────┘
```

Figure 4. Flow chart of data calibration scheme using homogeneous phantoms.

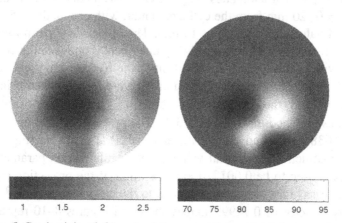

Figure 5. Conductivity (left) and relative permittivity (right) images of an agar phantom with a hole, recovered with the same system and concomitant measurement data that produced the images in Fig. 3. The data calibration scheme described in the text was used, eliminating the peripheral low-conductivity artifact and maintaining accuracy in the reconstructed property values. Units of conductivity image are S/m; relative permittivity is unitless.

6   THREE-DIMENSIONAL RECONSTRUCTION

In order to demonstrate 3D reconstruction capabilities, which are presently under development, we have used a cylindrical model of radius 50 mm and height 150 mm (Figure 6a). The mesh consisted of 10,295 nodes corresponding to 44,725 linear tetrahedral elements. Four planes of electrodes 30 mm apart were modeled, each plane consisting of 16 circular electrodes 5 mm in diameter. In order to ensure that equal numbers of nodes were used to model each electrode, their locations and shapes were taken into consideration during the meshing of the domain. The model was assigned the homogenous electrical properties $\sigma = 2$ S/m and $\varepsilon_r = 80$. All of the results presented here were confined to the excitation frequency of 125 kHz.

We have completed several studies using this model. In the first instance, the voltage drive mode was considered. In this mode, one applies a set of voltage patterns at all electrodes simultaneously and measures the resulting currents at all electrodes. Three current patterns were evaluated: (1) 15 sinusoidal current patterns over each plane, where all planes were in phase with each other; (2) 15 sinusoidal current patterns over each plane, where each plane was 45° out of phase with respect to its neighbors; and (3) 15 sinusoidal current patterns over each plane, where each plane was 90° out of phase with respect to its neighbors.

Boundary data were calculated for each set of current pattern in the presence of two spherical anomalies (Fig. 7). One was a conducting anomaly located at $z = 0$, 20 mm from the cylinder center, with conductivity 5 times the background value and a radius of 15 mm. The other was a permittive anomaly located at $z = 0$, 20 mm from the cylinder center opposite the conductive anomaly, with relative permittivity 10 times the background value and a radius of 15 mm. Using these data sets, images were reconstructed using a dual mesh scheme with the discretizations shown in Figure 6 (see discussion of the dual mesh method in Ch. 2, Sec. 3.2). The property estimation mesh consisted of 4638 nodes and 22,808 linear tetrahedral elements (Fig. 6b). For image reconstruction, the initial value of the regularization parameter λ in (5.13) was chosen to be 0.001. At each iteration, if the projection error, χ^2, was found to have decreased as compared to the last iteration then λ was decreased by a factor of 0.7499. Images shown in Figures 8–10 represent the 29th iteration, which was chosen because beyond this point χ^2 did not decrease by more than 0.1% from the previous iteration.

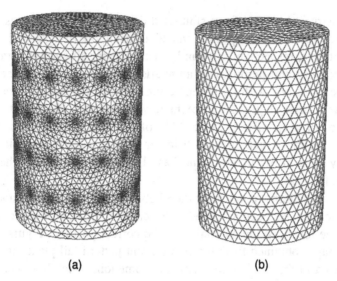

(a)   (b)

Figure 6. (a) Finite element model used for the generation of the Jacobian and synthetic measurement data for the 3D simulation experiments described in the text. The forward mesh is cylindrical with radius 50 mm and height 150 mm. Four planes of electrodes are modeled (at $z = -45$, -15, 15, and 45 mm), each plane containing 16 equally-spaced circular electrodes of radius 5 mm. (b) Finite element mesh used as the reconstruction basis. This mesh has the same geometrical dimensions as the field solution mesh in (a), but fewer degrees of freedom (nodes).

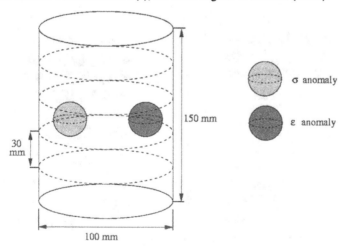

Figure 7. Schematic of the simulation model used to generate synthetic anomaly data for numerical experiments. Background conductivity and relative permittivity are 2 S/m and 80, respectively. As shown, a spherical conductive anomaly with conductivity 10 S/m and radius 15 mm is placed 20 mm left of the center at $z = 0$ mm, and a spherical permittivity anomaly with relative permittivity 800 and radius 15 mm is placed 20 mm right of the center at $z = 0$ mm.

Reconstructed images from simulated data with anomalies present in the domain are presented in Figures 8, 9, and 10 using the first, second, and third current patterns, respectively. It can be seen that for all current patterns both the conductivity and permittivity anomalies have been reconstructed in the correct locations and with good separation between the two physical properties. These images required approximately 10 minutes of computation time per iteration on a 1.7 GHz PC with 2 GB of RAM. It is evident that the property values in the targets are much lower than expected, a problem that is commonly seen in 3D imaging and has also been reported in other similar modalities [12, 13].

Using all patterns, good separation between the conductivity and permittivity anomalies has been achieved. Furthermore, although the reconstructed images have localized the anomalies in the correct position, Figure 11 shows that the images obtained from the first current pattern (all planes in-phase) is more blurred in the z direction. This phenomenon, which has been reported elsewhere, is a common problem in 3D imaging that is sometimes referred to as the "partial volume effect." Quantitative accuracy can be improved by using other types of regularization or reconstruction bases and by the addition of constraints or other *a priori* information.

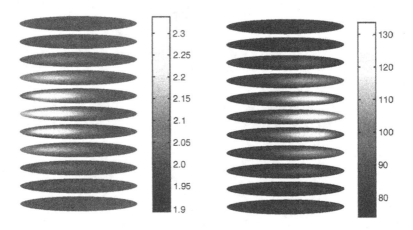

Figure 8. Simultaneously reconstructed images of conductivity (left) and relative permittivity (right) from data simulated using the first current drive pattern (i.e., in-phase pattern along the cylinder axis). Images represent the 29th iteration. Each image consists of cross-sections through the cylindrical model stacked at appropriate z levels to outline the cylinder. Conductivity grayscale units are S/m.

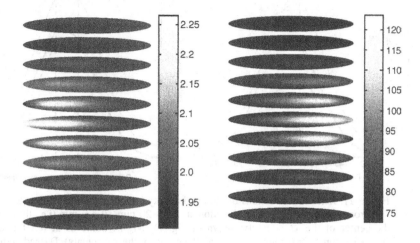

Figure 9. Same as Figure 8 (conductivity image on left, permittivity image on right) but using the second current drive pattern, i.e., each electrode plane 45° out of phase with its neighbors. Conductivity grayscale units are S/m.

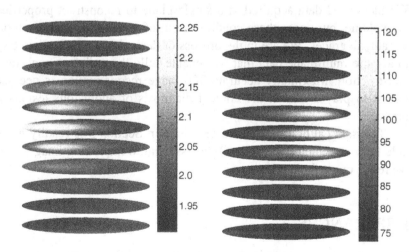

Figure 10. Same as Figures 8 and 9 (conductivity image on left, permittivity image on right) but using the third current drive pattern, i.e., each electrode plane 90° out of phase with its neighbors. Conductivity grayscale units are S/m.

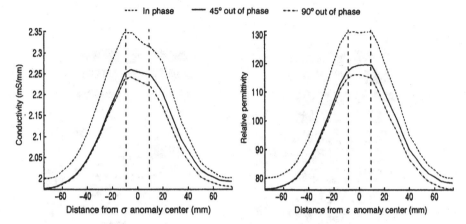

Figure 11. Left: Cross-sections of the conductivity images shown in Figures 8–10. The cross-sections are in the z direction at $x = -20$ mm, $y = 0$ mm (i.e., through the center of the σ anomaly shown in Fig. 7). *Right:* Same as at left but at $x = +20$ mm, $y = 0$ mm (i.e., through the center of the ε anomaly). Dashed vertical lines indicate the boundaries of the inclusion in each case (15 mm diameter).

7   CONCLUSION

We have used data acquired in a single plane to reconstruct properties in a 3D volume, but under these conditions out-of-plane structural resolution inevitably degrades. We are in the process of designing a new hardware system to acquire multiplane data that will enable fully three-dimensional image reconstruction. Maximally accurate 3D image reconstruction is necessary if EIS is to play a role in the clinical diagnosis of anomalous lesions in the breast.

The data calibration scheme described in Section 5 is readily generalizable to three dimensions, and will be essential to improving image quality as we refine our techniques.

REFERENCES

[1]   J. J. Ackmann and M. A. Seitz, "Methods of complex impedance measurements in biologic tissue." *CRC Crit. Rev. Biomed. Eng.*, Vol. 11, 1984, pp. 281–311.

[2]   E. Gersing and M. Osypka, "On the frequency range necessary for a multi-frequency tomograph." *Innov. Tech. Biol. Med.*, Vol. 15, 1994, pp. 70–71.

[3]   J. Jossinet, "Variability of impedivity in normal and pathological breast tissue." *Med. & Biol. Eng. & Comput.*, Vol. 34, 1996, pp. 346–350.

[4]   D. C. Barber and B. H. Brown, "Imaging spatial distribution of resistivity using applied potential tomography." *Electronics Lett.*, Vol. 19, 1983, 933–935.

[5]   A. Surowiec et al., "Dielectric properties of breast carcinoma and the surrounding tissues." *IEEE Trans. BME.*, Vol. 35, 1988, pp. 256–263.

[6]   L. M. Newcomer et al., "Detection method and breast carcinoma histology." *Cancer*, Vol. 95, 2002, pp. 470–477.

[7]   N. Polydorides and W. R. B. Lionheart, "A Matlab toolkit for three-dimensional impedance tomography: A contribution to the Electrical Impedance and Diffuse Optical Reconstruction Software Project." *Meas. Sci. Tech.*, Vol. 13, 2002, pp. 1871–1883.

[8]   M. T. Markova, *10 MHz Electrical Impedance Spectroscopy System.* Ph.D. dissertation, Thayer School of Engineering, Dartmouth College, Hanover, NH, 2002.

[9]   D. Isaacson, "Distinguishability of conductivities by electric current computed tomography." *IEEE Trans. Med. Imag.*, Vol. MI-5, 1986, pp. 91–95.

[10]   T. E. Kerner, *Electrical Impedance Tomography for Breast Imaging.* Ph.D. thesis, Thayer School of Engineering, Dartmouth College, Hanover, NH, June 2001.

[11]   N. K. Soni, H. Dehghani, A. Hartov, K. D. Paulsen, "A novel data calibration scheme for electrical impedance tomography." *Physiol. Meas.*, Vol. 24, 2003, 421–435.

[12]   H. Dehghani et al., "Multiwavelength three-dimensional near-infrared tomography of the breast: Initial simulation, phantom, and clinical results." *App. Opt.*, Vol. 42, 2003, pp. 135–145.

[13]   A. Gibson et al., "Optical tomography of a realistic neonatal head phantom." *App. Opt.*, Vol. 42(1), 2003.

Chapter 6

ELECTRICAL IMPEDANCE SPECTROSCOPY: TRANSLATION TO CLINIC

Alex Hartov, Ph.D., Ryan J. Halter, and Todd E. Kerner, M.D., Ph.D.

1   INTRODUCTION

This chapter describes our experience in building three generations of electrical impedance spectroscopy (EIS) systems. X-ray mammography, the currently accepted method for breast-cancer screening, has significant false-negative and false-positive rates, which lead to unnecessary biopsies; there is thus motivation for exploring EIS, among other modalities, as an alternative or complement to x-ray mammography.

The underlying rationale for using EIS in breast cancer screening is that significant differences between the electrical properties of malignant and normal breast tissues have been observed [1]. These differences are frequency-dependent. Greater differences in conductivity (σ) are seen at higher frequencies and greater differences in permittivity (ε) at lower frequencies.

2   GENERAL CONSIDERATIONS

Before describing the design and construction of our EIS systems, we clarify a few aspects and limitations of the technology. First, the spatial resolution and sensitivity of EIS are not uniform, but are greatest in the vicinity of the electrodes. This is directly related to the current distribution in the medium being interrogated, which is densest near the sourcing electrodes. As a result, the lowest spatial resolution and sensitivity will be observed in the central region of any cross-section (assuming that the electrodes are located around the periphery). Second, unpredictable contact-impedance variations between electrodes degrade image quality. Spatial resolution can be improved by using more electrodes; sensitivity to impedance variations can be improved by making the electrodes as large as possible, thus covering as much of the periphery as possible. Another way to improve sensitivity is to use the largest allowable current. In clinical applications, however, current is limited by patient safety considerations. In some situations (though not in breast imaging) it is possible to improve spatial resolution near a target subvolume by using internal electrodes.

EIS was first developed as a two-dimensional imaging technology. Image reconstructions were based on a number of assumptions. One—which is inherent to two-dimensional EIS, regardless of the method of image reconstruction adopted (e.g., back-projection or finite element)—is that current flows only in the imaging plane. Yet this clearly cannot be the case. For example, in a homogeneous cylindrical volume encircled by an array of electrodes set in a horizontal transecting plane, significant currents (i.e., currents that will have an impact on the measurements) will flow in a prolate spheroidal volume extending approximately half of the radius of the cylinder above and below the transecting plane. Impedance inhomogeneities that do not intersect the imaging plane can thus influence reconstructed 2D images by interacting with the current field. This is verifiable experimentally using high-contrast inclusions in a saline tank. For this reason, a fully three-dimensional treatment of the data is theoretically liable to produce better reconstruction results. This is true for data acquired both from a single planar array of electrodes and from three-dimensional arrays (e.g., multiple planar arrays).

3   FIRST-GENERATION SYSTEM *IN VITRO*

Having implemented the image-reconstruction algorithms described in the previous chapter, we realized a two-dimensional first-generation EIS system [2, 3]. The physical interface consisted of a shallow, circular, saline-filled tank in which conducting and insulating targets could be placed for imaging (Figure 1). The tank, 20 cm in diameter and 6 cm deep (filled to 4 cm depth with a 0.9% NaCl solution), was fabricated from a PVC pipe and mounted on a Lucite base. The 32 electrodes around the perimeter of the shallow tank were steel paper clips attached over the tank edge so that a portion of the wire (immersed area approximately 8.8×10^{-5} m^2) extended straight to the tank base. The goal was to create a simple platform on which to test the electronics and software, which could then be ported to a second-generation system with an electrode interface suitable for clinical breast imaging.

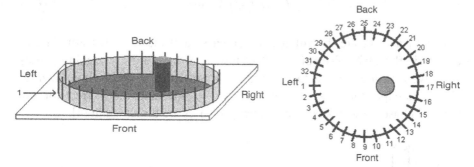

Figure 1. In vitro application of our first-generation, 32-electrode EIS system. The tank is depicted with a cylindrical target placed upright midway between electrode 17 and the tank's center.

We designed this system to provide maximum flexibility. Each channel could be operated in either voltage or current mode, with a relay switching either a voltage source or current source to the electrode as desired. The electrodes were driven by 32 in-phase sinusoidal signals at one of 10 selectable frequencies (10, 20, 40, 50, 70, 125, 225, 525, 750, and 950 kHz) supplied by a digitally-controlled source having 12-bit accuracy over a ±12 V, ±50 mA range (Datel PC-420, Mansfield, MA). All electrodes were excited and measured simultaneously, sampling being performed with a 16-bit, 200 kHz A/D board (Datel PCI-416M). Trigonometric excitation patterns were used, as was undersampling (to extend the effective bandwidth of the A/D board [3]). The system was controlled by a 200 MHz Pentium II PC via a 32-bit digital I/O board (DIO48, Cyber Research, Branford, CT). A simplified schematic of the electronics associated with a single channel is shown in Figure 2.

Calibration of system outputs and inputs was performed by a computerized utility using a special relay board that could individually connect each of the 32 channels to a known load [2, 4]. Our A/D board was calibrated using manufacturer specifications, while our waveform generator (the source of V_{ref}, Fig. 2) was calibrated by comparing the requested output to the output actually delivered (using the A/D board to measure the delivered output). The D/A in each channel (Fig. 2) was also calibrated by comparing requested to delivered outputs. Finally, precision loads were connected under computer control to the channels at their board connections. By using several load values, we characterized the relationship between the voltages and load currents across each channel's 100 Ω sense resistor. We then performed a three-parameter, two-dimensional, first-order linear regression of the form

$$I = \alpha V_1 + \beta V_2 + \gamma \tag{6.1}$$

where V_1 and V_2 are the voltages on either side of the sense resistor (Fig. 2) and γ is the residual error or offset term. Furthermore, by making phase-sensitive measurements with reactive loads consisting of precisely-known resistor and capacitor networks we were able to determine and correct for any channel phase skew. System performance metrics are discussed in [4].

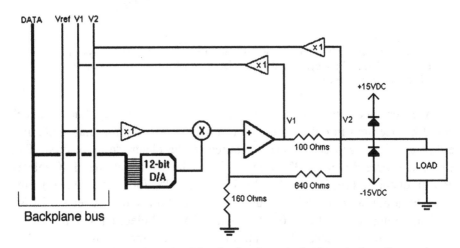

Figure 2. Simplified schematic of the circuitry for a single channel of our first- and second-generation EIS systems. V_1 and V_2 are sampled by the A/D board, not shown. V_{ref} is a reference sinusoid sent to all channels. The load includes both electrode and target. Circuitry is shown only for the voltage mode; current mode is achieved by disconnecting the OP amp, 640-Ω resistor, and 160-Ω resistor from the circuit and replacing them with a current source connected between the mixer output (i.e., the + input of the OP amp) and V_1. Relays and control lines are omitted from this drawing.

We did not measure signal magnitude and phase in hardware. Rather, in order to achieve affordable lock-in performance over the relatively wide frequency range of the system, our channel circuits were designed to sample the AC voltage across a sense resistor in series with the electrode. A software lock-in amplifier algorithm was then used to extract signal magnitude and phase from the data.

We began by imaging a wide range of targets consisting of conducting (brass) and nonconducting (nylon) cylinders of various diameters placed upright at various points in the tank. We acquired data for each target at all 10 frequencies, which took approximately 3.5 min. Usually we recorded two signal periods at 101 samples/period. Representative *in vitro* results are shown in Figure 3.

Blurring of feature borders, as seen in Figure 3, is an artifact of the reconstruction algorithm, in which the final value at each property mesh node is a function of the values at all other nodes. An electrode-associated peripheral artifact is also apparent (top row). As discussed in the previous chapter, numerical electrode modeling only slightly reduces the latter artifact; difference imaging does so more effectively. In difference imaging, the absolute node values in a target image are subtracted from those calculated for a homogeneous tank. Amelioration of peripheral artifact in the saline-tank setup by means of difference imaging is indicated in Figure 3, which compares absolute and difference images of a 0.64 cm diameter conducting cylinder at three depths. The contact impedances for the saline-immersed electrodes in the two-dimensional tank geometry were nearly invariant and identical, providing optimal conditions, but difference imaging does not cope equally well with nonuniform contact impedances, which occur clinically.

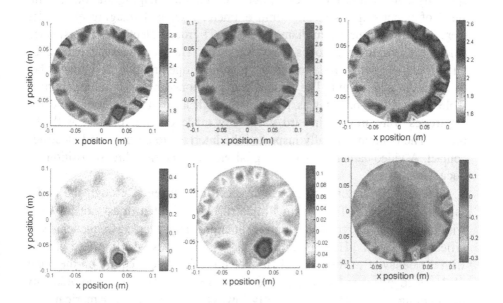

Figure 3. Absolute (upper row) and difference (lower row) conductivity images of a 0.64-cm-diameter brass cylinder placed 1 cm (left), 2 cm (center), and 4 cm (right) from electrode 10 (at about 5 o'clock). Images were acquired in voltage mode at 950 kHz. Graybar units are S/m.

Using the saline-tank configuration, we verified that electrode artifact is less pronounced at higher frequencies and characterized system resolution as a function of inclusion width and distance from the center of the imaging region [1, 2]. We found that conductors are distinguishable at greater depth than insulators of equal size, though difference imaging improves maximum resolvable depth for both types of targets. The effect of difference imaging on the depth resolution of a conducting target is evident in Figure 3. Resolvability diminishes with target depth for both the absolute and difference images, but more slowly for the difference images. The target used in Figure 3 was essentially undetectable at depths greater than 4 cm, even in difference images. A conducting target had to be greater than 2.5 cm in diameter to be detected at the center of the tank.

4   FIRST-GENERATION SYSTEM *IN VIVO*

To render our first-generation system suitable for clinical use, we employed a specially-constructed electrode system and patient imaging station [5]. Instead of paper clips, sixteen 8 mm diameter Ag/AgCl imaging electrodes were used (plus four 4 mm diameter Ag/AgCl ground electrodes interspersed among the imaging electrodes at 90° intervals). The electrodes were mounted on radially adjustable rods to create an annular opening with a diameter between 5 cm and 18 cm. The patient was positioned prone on an examining table so that one breast was pendant through a circular opening, and the electrodes were moved inward until they made circular contact with the breast. The operator visually inspected the interface to ensure good electrode contact. A video camera provided digital views of the final breast position for documentation.

Because EIS intentionally passes electrical currents through the body, safety is a concern. The currents injected by the system must not interfere with any normal electrophysiological functions. However, at frequencies significantly above 1 kHz it is unlikely that AC currents will interfere grossly with the behavior of ion channels in the cell wall, which require on the order of 1 ms to open and close; furthermore, resistive heating is avoided by maintaining current flow sufficiently low. Our system meets American National Standards Institute guidelines for maximum current as a function of frequency (ANSI/AAMI ES1-1993). Further, the EIS system is electrically isolated from earth ground through the use of an isolating transformer. This prevents possible return-current paths through grounded objects. Currents can enter and leave the body only via the imaging electrodes.

After testing the new electrode system on agar and fruit phantoms and on the arm and leg [2], we undertook clinical exams of the breast. In a preliminary study of 12 volunteers having among them 14 abnormal breasts (i.e., breasts containing lesions identified as suspicious by mammography), 11 (79%) of the abnormal breasts were correctly identified by inspection of EIS images, all four (100%) of the tumors present were identified, and 9 (82%) of the normal breasts were identified [6]. (Quantitative analysis of the images was also performed but had lower accuracy.) Images of a normal breast, a breast with cyst, and a breast with a large tumor are shown in Figure 4. In Figure 5, a complete set of conductivity and permittivity images are shown for the cystic breast in Figure 4 and the contralateral breast of the same individual.

We conducted additional studies of 26 women in 2001–2002 using a second-generation breast interface with improved electrode-positioning control [7]. Using trigonometric excitation patterns, we acquired voltage-mode images at the 10 frequencies listed in the previous section. Breasts designated as abnormal on the basis of preliminary mammograms were imaged in three planes: one above the level of the suspicious lesion, one at the level of the lesion, and one below the level of the lesion. The image-reconstruction algorithm was executed for five iterations in each case. Images from the five highest frequencies were judged visually for the presence of abnormalities, based on earlier reproducibility studies which showed that the most consistent images were generated at these frequencies.

Fifty-one breasts were imaged in this study. These included 38 normal breasts and six containing ACR 4 or 5 lesions.* Thirty (79%) of the normal breasts and five (83%) of the ACR 4 or 5 breasts were correctly identified by visual inspection of our EIS images. These provisional results show a rate of cancer detection comparable to that achieved by groups using surface-impedance mapping methods [7], but it is notable the latter approaches are intrinsically limited to depths of a few centimeters, whereas our tomographic technique has the potential to resolve abnormalities near the center of the imaging volume.

---

* In the American College of Radiology (ACR) BI-RADS rating system, ACR 1 is negative; ACR2 is a benign finding, negative; ACR 3 is probably a benign finding; ACR 4 is a suspicious abnormality; and ACR 5 is highly suggestive of malignancy (American College of Radiology, *Breast Imaging Reporting and Date System* (*BI-RADS*), 3rd Edition, Reston, VA, 1998).

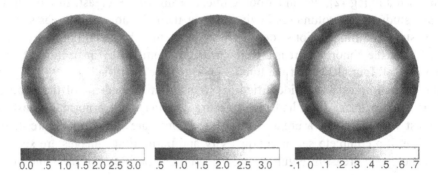

0.0 .5 1.0 1.5 2.0 2.5 3.0   .5   1.0 1.5 2.0 2.5 3.0   -.1 0 .1 .2 .3 .4 .5 .6 .7

Figure 4. Three clinical images from our first-generation EIS system. *Left*: Normal breast. *Center*: Breast with a cyst (bright area at 3 o'clock). *Right*: breast with a large tumor (elliptical bright area dominating the superior portion of the image from 10 to 3 o'clock). These are voltage-mode images acquired at 125 kHz. Graybar units are S/m.

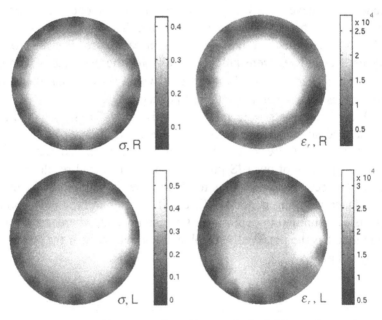

Figure 5. Images from a subject presenting with a cyst in the left breast (bottom image pair in Fig. 4). *Left*: Conductivity (σ) images for right (R) and left (L) breasts (units S/m). *Right*: relative permittivity (ε_r) images for right and left breasts (dimensionless).

5   SECOND- AND THIRD-GENERATION SYSTEMS

5.1   Design Overview

Our first-generation EIS system suffered from two fundamental limitations. The first was its two-dimensionality. As noted above, during impedance tomography of a three-dimensional target some current will inevitably traverse out-of-plane regions, distorting two-dimensional images. Combining data acquired sequentially at multiple planes does not enable three-dimensional imaging per se because the breast deforms under pressure, producing a different geometry when the data is acquired in each plane. Optimization of a three-dimensional finite element model using two-dimensional data, though possible, suffers from having too few data points to meaningfully adjust so many degrees of freedom.

The second limitation of our first-generation system was its bandwidth. Experience showed that the best images were generally obtained at the highest available operating frequency (950 kHz), which was consistent with various studies arguing that frequencies above 1 MHz are better for the bioelectrical characterization of various types of tissue in the breast [8–10]. Higher frequencies were thus desirable.

We planned our second-generation system to acquire data simultaneously in multiple planes and to operate at any frequency between 10 kHz and 10 MHz [11]. Extension to high frequencies entails problems with stray capacitance, signal generation, and signal sampling. To bring the driving and sensing electronics as close as possible to the electrodes, we integrated custom-built circuit boards with the breast interface. Each board contained the sampling and driving circuitry for a pair of channels. Each channel was configured under computer control to sample the voltage across a sense resistor or to drive the electrode in voltage or current mode. The boards were wedge-shaped to allow placement of all electronics components as close as possible to the electrodes. Sixteen such boards were arranged around a radially-adjustable array of 16 electrodes similar to that used in our first-generation system. Use of 32 channels allowed for simultaneous driving and measurement on all 16 electrodes. Up to four such 32-channel, 16-electrode levels could, in principle, be stacked to enable three-dimensional imaging, but we did not construct a multilevel system using our second-generation hardware design.

We gained valuable experience from our second-generation system, and it has been retained for *in vitro* studies. However, the integration times required by the analog RMS-to-DC converters and phase detectors that employed in this system (as opposed to the software lock-in amplifier solution we used in our first-generation system) resulted in longer examination times than were acceptable for patient studies. Design details of our second-generation system are therefore omitted here in favor of those of our third-generation system, which is now being used clinically.

Our third-generation system consists of four stacked annular arrays with 16 electrodes in each plane. Radially arranged wedge-shaped circuit boards are used, as in the second-generation design, but perform signal control, generation, and processing using digital signal processor (DSP) technology. This reduces the analog signal path for each channel to a minimum (less than 10 cm) and allows arbitrary waveform generation.

Individual wedge boards contain the circuitry for four bidirectional channels, with each stackable layer comprising eight wedge boards. A dedicated custom-built control board allows the user interface computer (a 1.79 GHz AMD Athlon™ laptop) to interact with the wedge boards and mechanical electrode-positioning system for each layer. The basic layout for a single layer is shown in Figure 6. An individual wedge board and three stacked layers are shown in Figure 7.

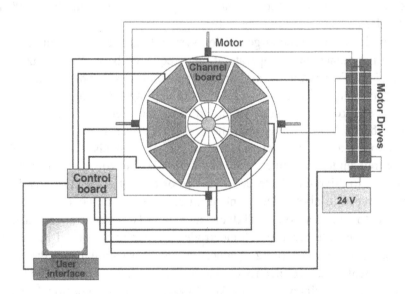

Figure 6. System layout for a single 32-channel layer of our third-generation EIS system. The system may be configured with one to four layers. Each layer has its own control board. Each motor moves four electrodes in a single layer.

As in previous systems, the breast interface is placed under an examination table below the opening into which the breast is introduced (Fig. 8). Electrode position is adjusted radially at each level (5–18 cm adjustable opening diameter) to enable the electrodes to make contact with the breast. The height (distance from the chest wall) of each level is fixed, the first level being approximately 1.5 cm from the chest wall and the following levels 3 cm apart. This multilevel configuration makes it possible to acquire planar data at multiple levels for reconstruction of multiple two-dimensional images or to acquire data on all levels simultaneously for reconstruction of three-dimensional images. From the channel-design point of view, the 2D/3D distinction is not crucial except that three-dimensional imaging implies more channels.

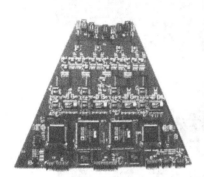 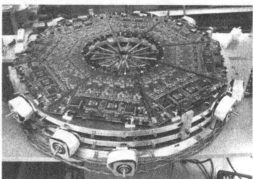

Figure 7. Left: A four-channel board in our third-generation EIS system. *Right*: A stack of three eight-board layers with the top mechanical layer removed. Each layer is 60 cm in diameter. The round protrusions in the photograph at right are the motors that adjust electrode position (four motors per layer). The control boards and user-interface computer do not appear in the picture.

5.2   Channel Board Design and Signal Processing

We found that the best way to generate and measure signals up to 10 MHz while still maintaining a compact design was to incorporate a combination of advanced DSP chips, reconfigurable logic devices (field programmable gate arrays [FPGAs]), high-performance digital-to-analog converters (DACs), and analog-to-digital converters (ADCs). The DSP chip we use is a 32-bit ADSP-21065L (Analog Devices, Norwood, MA), clocked at 66 MHz; the FPGA is a XILINX Spartan XC2S30™ (XILINX, San Jose, CA) clocked as high as 80 MHz; the DAC is a 14-bit AD9754 (Analog Devices); and the ADC is a 16-bit differential AD7677AST (Analog Devices) with a maximum through-

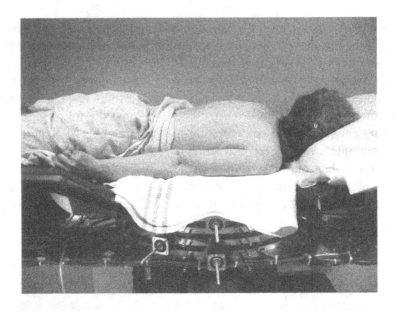

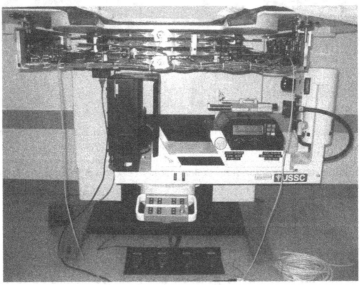

Figure 8. Third-generation EIS patient-imaging station. *Top*: Subject prone on table with four-level breast interface partly visible below. *Bottom*: Breast interface presented in profile view. The shield that normally covers the mechanical and electronics assemblies has been removed for illustration. A standard x-ray biopsy table has been adapted by mounting two rails on its underside, allowing the EIS assembly to slide in and out like a drawer. The x-ray unit and detector assembly for a biopsy procedure remain in place. Moving the x-ray components as low as possible with respect to the table leaves a 7.5" gap that is sufficient for mounting the EIS imaging system.

put of 1 million samples per second. The applied voltage range is 4 V peak-to-peak. A simplified schematic of a single channel is shown in Figure 9.

We use a dual-ported pattern memory (implemented in the FPGA) to create the applied signal. Bits 0–13 of the 256×16 pattern memory in the FPGA are fed to a 14-bit DAC; this is followed by a buffer stage to create the applied signal, while bit 14 is used to trigger the ADCs that sample V_1 and V_2, the voltages on both sides of the sensing resistor R_s. This allows sampling to take place in lockstep with signal generation.

Signal frequency is established by a combination of the number of words that make up a full signal cycle in the pattern memory, *nwords*, and the signal memory clock, F_{clock}: that is, $F_{sig} = F_{clock} / nwords$. With this arrangement, the extensive range of frequencies targeted for this design is readily achievable. A few exemplary configurations are listed in Table 1.

All channels are controlled by a common clock, with a channel timing skew of less than 2 ns. The pattern clock is produced by a direct-digital-synthesis chip on a control board that communicates with all channel boards. The DSP chip executes at 66 MHz asynchronously with respect to the pattern clock. Its interaction with the ADCs is interrupt-driven. The DSP chip computes the pattern values based on the requested amplitude and frequency, then loads them into the pattern RAM. It also collects the measured values from both ADCs, and from these computes V_{Re}, V_{Im}, I_{Re}, and I_{Im} for a given electrode. These four floating-point values are then sent to the controller, which in turn relays the information to the system computer.

Computation of the complex AC values of V and I by the DSP chip is a two-step process. The first step converts the 16-bit integer data from the ADCs into voltages. This is accomplished using a calibration curve obtained by using the ADCs to measure DC voltages that are simultaneously recorded with a trusted precision instrument. A linear regression is computed between the known voltages and the ADC numerical values to obtain slope and offset calibration parameters.

The second step computes the complex values from the measurements. Two techniques are available to perform vector (i.e., real and imaginary or magnitude and phase) voltage measurements, namely, quadrature sampling and mixing. In quadrature sampling, two samples are recorded per cycle of the measured waveform. Since acquisition timing occurs in lockstep with the waveform generator, we place samples at the first positive peak and the following zero crossing of the input waveform. These samples correspond to the 0° and 90° phase points in the waveform. The measured values correspond to the waveform's real and imaginary components, the phase being

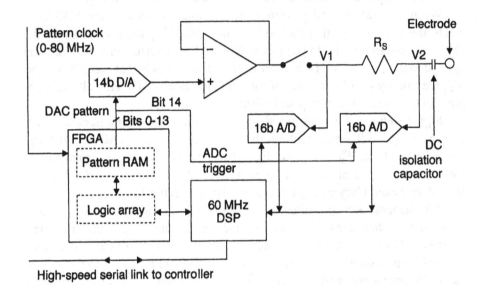

Figure 9. Simplified schematic of a single DSP-based channel in our third-generation EIS system. Drawing shows half of a two-channel circuit in which both channels share the FPGA and the DSP controller. Each wedge board contains two dual-channel circuits for a total of four channels per board. Compare to the channel schematic for our second-generation system (Fig. 2).

F_{sig} (Hz)	npoints	F_{clock} (MHz)
10,000	256	2.560
21,544	256	5.515
46,416	256	11.882
100,000	256	25.600
215,443	256	55.154
464,159	172	79.714
1,000,000	80	80.000
2,154,435	37	79.714
4,641,589	17	78.907
10,000,000	8	80.000

Table 1. Relationship between pattern memory clock and various applied signal frequencies (based on an FPGA memory depth of 256 words).

referenced to the input waveform. From this information, any representation of the AC waveform sampled can be computed. Given the in-phase and quadrature voltages V_i and V_q, we have

$$|V| = \sqrt{V_i^2 + V_q^2}, \quad \theta_v = \arctan\left(\frac{V_q}{V_i}\right), \quad \text{Re}(V) = V_i, \quad \text{and} \quad \text{Im}(V) = V_q. \quad (6.2)$$

Mixing, on the other hand, requires that the signal be sampled at multiple points, not just two. The real and imaginary parts of the signal are obtained by mixing the signal samples with synthetic (i.e., computed) sine and cosine waveforms. Assuming that the zero-phase reference signal is a cosine, the products of mixing with the synthetic sine and cosine waveforms will be the real and imaginary components, respectively, of the measured signal. The mixing operation itself consists of multiplying the signal samples with the synthetic waveform samples and averaging:

$$\text{Re}(V) = \frac{1}{N}\sum_{i=1}^{N} V_{cos}(i) \cdot V_{sig}(i), \quad \text{Im}(V) = \frac{1}{N}\sum_{i=1}^{N} V_{sin}(i) \cdot V_{sig}(i),$$

$$|V| = \sqrt{\text{Re}(V)^2 + \text{Im}(V)^2}, \quad \text{and} \quad \theta_v = \arctan\left(\frac{\text{Im}(V)}{\text{Re}(V)}\right). \quad (6.3)$$

We sample V_1 and V_2 (see Fig. 9) but seek the complex-valued electrode voltage and current, with the phase of the load current I_L expressed with respect to the load voltage V_L. For this reconstruction, we need $\text{Re}(V_L)$, $\text{Im}(V_L)$, $\text{Re}(I_L)$, and $\text{Im}(I_L)$. V_2 will have some phase skew due to the buffer OP amp and the impedance in series with the driver. This phase can be removed by rotating the V_2 phasor in the phase plane to the $0°$ position. V_L and I_L can then be found from the following relationships:

$$\text{Re}(V_L) = |V_2|, \quad \text{Im}(V_L) = 0, \quad I = \frac{(V_1 - V_2)}{R_s},$$

$$\theta_{V2} = \arctan\left(\frac{\text{Im}(V_2)}{\text{Re}(V_2)}\right), \quad \theta_I = \arctan\left(\frac{\text{Im}(I)}{\text{Re}(I)}\right),$$

$$\text{Re}(I_L) = \frac{|V_1 - V_2|}{R_s}\cos(\theta_I - \theta_{V_2}),$$

$$\text{and} \quad \text{Im}\left(I_L\right) = \left| \frac{V_1 - V_2}{R_s} \right| \sin\left(\theta_I - \theta_{V_2}\right). \tag{6.4}$$

Debate exists over whether it is preferable to apply currents or voltages and then measure the resulting voltages or currents. In the design presented here, the driver circuitry falls into the voltage-mode category. However, by programming the DSP appropriately one can use the channel as a current source. This is achieved by measuring the current in real time and applying an adjusted scaling factor to the signal pattern data to produce the desired levels.

5.3   Three-Dimensional Trigonometric Excitation

As discussed in the previous chapter, trigonometric signal patterns are optimal for two-dimensional imaging of a circularly symmetric target. Our new system raises the question of the optimal signaling scheme in *three* dimensions. We have conjectured that spatially rotating the trigonometric signal patterns in the third (vertical) dimension will be close to optimal. In effect, in a four-level system we apply a spatial rotation of 90° to the trigonometric pattern for each successive layer (Fig. 10). We have not yet compared this pattern to others experimentally.

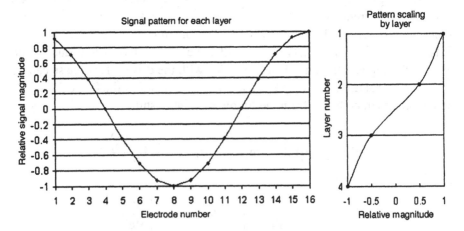

Figure 10. Three-dimensional trigonometric excitation scheme. *Left*: Pattern applied to the 16 electrodes of a single layer. *Right*: Pattern applied to a four-layer system. Continuous curves show ideal variation, points show actual (discrete) values.

It should be noted that trigonometric patterns are only optimal for homogeneous domains. For practical applications, optimality will depend on the spatial distribution of the load. Algorithms have been presented [12] which iteratively estimate the optimal patterns for a given load. Another approach would be to use vectors with random magnitudes, as explained in [13].

5.4   Breast Interface

The breast interface is one of the most critical components of an EIS system, as poor electrode contact will result in poor images. Further, image reconstruction requires precise knowledge of the relative positions of the electrodes in space. Some EIS groups approximate electrode position by a circular geometry even when the arrangement is clearly not circular, the electrodes being attached to a patient's chest, for example. As breasts are easily deformed, we have the opportunity to shape the imaged volume into a circular cross section. The electrodes have been configured in a circular array of adjustable diameter (Fig. 11); by bringing them into contact with the breast, we deform it into a circular shape. Only mild pressure is required and there is no discomfort to the patient. In contrast, many women avoid mammograms because they find the required breast compression uncomfortable and in some instances painful [15].

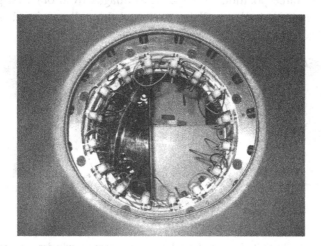

Figure 11. View of third-generation system looking straight down through the hole in the examining table. Electrodes are retracted as far as they will go. A two-layer system configuration was in place when this photograph was taken. See Fig. 8 for two side views of the patient-imaging station as a whole.

An additional clinical advantage of our new system is its speed of operation. The high-speed serial port interface we have used to interconnect the system interface computer, the control modules, and the channel modules offers the possibility of data acquisition at near-video rate: a 4-layer, 10-frequency exam will take about 1 minute. Postprocessing of the data to produce images requires considerably more time.

5.5   Preliminary Results

We have performed phantom studies and pilot breast exams with our third-generation system, but the hardware is still being calibrated and optimized and extensive results will take some months to acquire and analyze. We expect, however, to realize a significant increase in diagnostic capability over earlier systems due to the increased precision and dimensionality of the new system.

Figure 12 shows some of the results of a recently completed phantom study. We suspended a brass cylinder 1.3 cm in diameter in three positions in a saline tank and acquired data from a single electrode plane at 1.129 MHz. (Data were also acquired at 127.4 kHz and 3.36 MHz, but are not shown.) Conductivity and permittivity images were reconstructed simultaneously using a two-dimensional finite element mesh with 1345 nodes and 2560 linear triangular elements. The clarity and consistency with which the anomaly is imaged at the three positions, compared to images from our first-generation system (see Fig. 3), bodes well for two- and three-dimensional imaging of more complex targets.

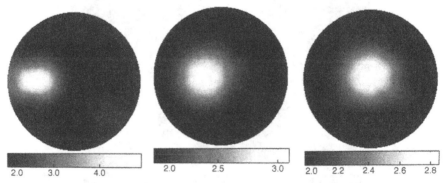

Figure 12. Conductivity images of a 1.3 cm–diameter brass cylinder suspended in a saline tank 8.5 cm across. The brass cylinder is shown 1 cm from tank's edge (left), 2 cm from the tank's edge (middle), and in the center of the tank (right). Images were acquired in voltage mode. Graybar units are S/m.

6   CONCLUSION

It is not expected that EIS will compete with x-rays, magnetic resonance imaging, or computerized tomography for image resolution. The available data suggests, however, that it may be more specific in discriminating between certain types of soft tissues, specifically in showing large contrast for malignant breast tissues as compared to normal breast or fat [1]. As a result, although reconstructed EIS images have relatively poor spatial resolution, certain types of small abnormalities leave a noticeable signature in the resulting images when compared to normal tissues.

With completion of our highly flexible third-generation EIS system this technology will have achieved a level of sophistication that may allow it to be used as an immediate follow-up to mammography when abnormalities are observed. In such cases, it may help differentiate between malignant and benign observations.

REFERENCES

[1]   J. Jossinet, "The impedivity of freshly excised human breast tissue." *Phys. Meas.*, Vol. 19, 1998, pp. 61–75.

[2]   T. E. Kerner et al., "Electrical impedance imaging at multiple frequencies in phantoms." *Physiol. Meas.*, Vol. 21, 2000, pp. 67–77.

[3]   T. E. Kerner, *Electrical Impedance Tomography for Breast Imaging*. Ph.D. Dissertation, Thayer School of Engineering, Dartmouth College, Hanover, NH, June, 2001.

[4]   D. B. Williams, *Characterization and Calibration of an Electrical Impedance Spectroscopy System*. Master's Thesis, Thayer School of Engineering, Dartmouth College, Hanover, NH, June, 1999.

[5]   A. Hartov et al., "A multichannel continuously selectable multifrequency electrical impedance spectroscopy measurement system." *IEEE Trans. Biomed. Eng.*, Vol. 47, 2000, pp. 49–57.

[6]   K. S. Osterman et al., "Multifrequency electrical impedance imaging: Preliminary in vivo experience in breast," *Physiol. Meas.*, Vol. 21, 2000, pp. 99–109.

[7]   T. E. Kerner et al., "Electrical impedance spectroscopy of the breast: Clinical imaging results in 26 subjects." *IEEE Trans. Med. Imag.*, Vol. 21, 2002, pp. 638–645.

[8]   E. Gersing and M. Osypka, "Tissue impedance spectra and the appropriate frequencies for EIT." *Physiol. Meas.*, Vol. 16, 1995, pp. A49–A55.

[9]   A. J. Surowiec et al., "Dielectric properties of breast carcinoma and the surrounding tissues," *IEEE Trans. Biomed. Engineering*, Vol.35, April 1988.

[10]   C. Gabriel, S. Gabriel, and E. Corthout, "The dielectric properties of biological tissues: I. Literature survey." *Phys. Med. Biol.*, Vol. 41, 1996, pp. 2231–2249.

[11]   M. T. Markova, *10 MHz Electrical Impedance Spectroscopy System*. Ph.D. dissertation, Thayer School of Engineering, Dartmouth College, Hanover, NH, 2002.

[12]   P. Hua et al., "Improved methods to determine optimal currents in electrical impedance tomography," *IEEE Trans. Med. Imag.*, Vol. 11, December, 1992.

[13] E. Demidenko et al., "On optimal current patterns for electrical impedance tomography." Submitted *IEEE Trans. Biomed. Eng.*, 2003.

[14] K. R. Foster, "Thermographic detection of breast cancer," *IEEE Eng. Med. Biol. Mag.*, Nov./Dec. 1998, pp. 10–14.

Chapter 7

MICROWAVE IMAGING: A MODEL-BASED APPROACH

Paul M. Meaney, Ph.D. and Qianqian Fang

1   INTRODUCTION

Microwave signals, which are nonionizing, tissue-penetrating, and focusable, are attractive for the diagnosis and treatment of various disorders, especially cancer. They have been used, for example, as a noninvasive means of delivering energy for the hyperthermic treatment of tumors [1, 2].

In the realm of diagnosis, microwave techniques are generally of two types, *backscatter* and *transmission* (or *tomographic*). Investigators have often sought to apply expertise gained with radar technology during the Cold War, with a resulting emphasis on backscatter techniques [3]. Backscatter is central to radar because the medium between antenna and target (vacuum or air) is essentially homogeneous and because targets are primarily in the far field of the antenna radiation pattern.

For medical diagnosis, however, the objects being interrogated (human bodies) are generally in the near field and therefore invite a different approach. The most common near-field technique is x-ray computed tomography (CT) [4]. In x-ray CT, signals are transmitted through the body from a large number of positions and detected on the opposite side. Because x-rays propagate in nearly straight lines through the body, are minimally scattered, and undergo absorption that is proportional to tissue density, high-resolution tomographic images can be produced using linear algorithms in which the value of each image pixel represents the radiodensity of a corresponding tissue volume. This approach has been used for diagnosis of conditions where tissue radiodensity is correlated to pathology. The method does have certain drawbacks, however, such as minimal sensitivity in certain situations (e.g., in detecting tumors that do not differ greatly in radiodensity from healthy tissue [5]). Further, x-rays expose patients to ionizing radiation, which carries a cumulatively increased risk of genetic damage [6].

Magnetic permeability is effectively uniform in the body, while permittivity and conductivity vary locally depending largely on water, fat, and protein content [7–10]. Generally, water molecules (which are highly polar) have high relative permittivity ranging from 79.7 at 300 MHz to 77.3 at 3 GHz. Water undergoes a molecular relaxation near 25 GHz, where its permittivity drops considerably.* The relative permittivity of fatty tissue and bone, which consist mostly of nonpolar molecules, ranges from 5 to 15 over this frequency band [8]. Further, water in the body is generally in the form of serum, whose main constituent is saline. Consequently, tissues with higher water content, such as muscle, have higher conductivity than fatty tissue or bone [12].

The variability of permittivity and conductivity within the body suggests that imaging of these properties in a noninvasive manner may have diagnostic value. Developing an imaging system in this frequency range has, however, been challenging [13–16], because microwaves, unlike x-rays, undergo significant reflection and refraction in the body. Figure 1 shows simulated two-dimensional electric-field magnitude contours for a microwave point source illuminating a circular, high-contrast target. Significant field variations occur both inside and outside the object. Further, in practice scattering occurs in *three* dimensions.

Other types of microwave breast imaging that are currently under investigation, though not discussed further in this text, include (1) confocal microwave approaches developed by Hagness et al. [17–19] and by Fear et al. [20–22], which seek to locate high-contrast objects without recovering their actual electrical properties; (2) passive radiometric techniques developed by Carr et al. [23] and Mouty et al. [24], which act to identify subsurface hot spots associated with tumor metabolism; (4) a thermoacoustic approach realized by Kruger et al. [25], which excites the breast tissue volume with a high-power microwave pulse and records the resulting microwave property-based mechanical displacements with an ultrasound transducer; and (4) other

---

* Note that we extend the lower bound of the "microwave" frequency range from its standard 1 GHz down to 300 MHz. Our definition preserves the standard wavelength range, not the standard frequency range; the wavelength used to define the standard bound is computed in free space ($\varepsilon_r = 1$ for vacuum), while the wavelength in a material medium is proportional to the free-space wavelength divided by the square root of the medium's relative permittivity [11].

microwave tomographic approaches reported by Bulyshev et al. [26] and Zhang et al. [27].

The rest of this chapter will discuss the algorithms involved in a two-dimensional microwave imaging system developed by our group with special attention to breast imaging. We begin below by describing the electric field with a truncated Taylor series [28]. This series forms the basis of an inverse, iterative, Newton-type numerical solution [29–31]. Next, we detail a forward solution for the electric field based on a hybrid numerical approach utilizing both finite element and boundary element methods [26, 32]. Finally, we cover several optimization issues. These include (1) choice of antenna-array elements [33]; (2) compensation for the presence of nonactive antenna elements [34, 35]; (3) log-magnitude/phase representation of the reconstruction algorithm [16] (especially useful when imaging large scatterers such as the

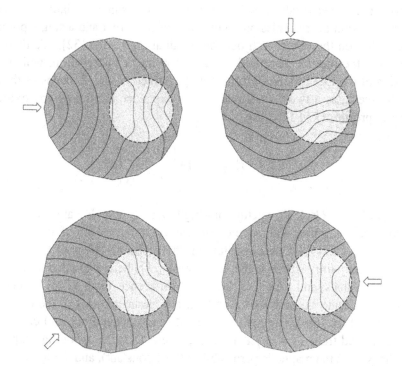

Figure 1. Calculated log-magnitude electric-field distributions within a circular imaging zone containing an off-center circular target (light area with dashed border). Four possible transmitter placements are shown. Field distribution is notably dependent on angle of illumination and distance to target.

breast; and (4) a conformal-mesh approach to improving property characterization of an object (e.g., breast) embedded in a homogeneous background (e.g., saline pool) [36]. Chapter 8 will discuss simulations and phantom experiments demonstrating overall system capability, along with clinical results from initial studies.

2   GAUSS-NEWTON IMAGE RECONSTRUCTION ALGORITHM

2.1   General Derivation

We first assume two finite element (FE) meshes covering the imaging zone, as described in Chapter 2: an N-point electric-field mesh and a coextensive L-node parameter mesh ($L < N$) [37]. We also assume, initially, that there is a single point of transmission on one side of the target and a single point of observation on the other, both outside the dual mesh area [32]. We then approximate the true electric field $\mathbf{E}_T$ at the point of observation, which is a function of the true property profile, $\{k_T^2\}$, defined on the L nodes of the parameter mesh, as a two-term Taylor series expanded around an approximate property profile, $\{k_A^2\}$ [26, 38]:

$$\mathbf{E}_T\left(\left\{k_T^2\right\}\right) \approx \mathbf{E}_A\left(\left\{k_A^2\right\}\right) + \left[\frac{\partial \mathbf{E}_A}{\partial k^2}\right]_A \left\{\Delta k^2\right\} \qquad (7.1)$$

Here $\{k_T^2\}$ and $\{k_A^2\}$ are vectors of length L; $\mathbf{E}_T$ and $\mathbf{E}_A$ are the true and approximate complex-valued electric fields at the point of observation; $[\partial \mathbf{E}_A / \partial k^2]$ is a $1 \times L$ matrix containing the first derivatives of the approximate solution with respect to the L variables, k_j^2, here evaluated at their approximate values; and $\{\Delta k^2\}$ is the vector difference $\{k_T^2\} - \{k_A^2\}$. When k_j^2 is given (j being the index of a node in the parameter mesh), the electrical properties at that node (i.e., permittivity ε_j and conductivity σ_j) can easily be determined from $k_j^2 = \omega^2 \mu \varepsilon_j + i\omega\mu\sigma_j$, where ω is the operating frequency in radians, μ is the magnetic permeability (here constant), and $i = \sqrt{-1}$.

The above relationship describes a single observable, that is, the electric field at a single point of observation (receiving antenna). The number of observables can be increased both by measuring the electric field produced by a single excitation (microwave transmission) at multiple points of observation and by providing excitations at different locations. The number of observations per image reconstruction, O_{IM}, is the product of the number of excitations, N_E, and the number of observations per excitation, O_E. (In our system, 16 antennas illuminate the imaging zone, allowing 16 distinct excitations and 15 observation points per excitation; hence, $N_E = 16$, $O_E = 15$, and $O_{IM} = 16 \times 15 = 240$.) For $O_{IM} > 1$, as in the image reconstruction problem, (7.1) becomes the matrix equation

$$\left[\; J \; \right]\left\{\Delta k^2\right\} = \left\{E_m\right\} - \left\{E_c\right\} \qquad (7.2)$$

where E_T in (7.1) has been replaced by the vector of actually measured electric field values, $\{E_m\}$, O_{IM} entries long; E_A has been replaced by the vector of calculated electric-field values, $\{E_c\}$; $\{\Delta k^2\}$ is L entries long; and the $O_{IM} \times L$ Jacobian matrix $[J]$ equals $[\partial E_c / \partial k^2]$. A least-squares fit for $\{\Delta k^2\}$ is obtained by solving the set of normal equations produced by multiplying of both sides of (7.2) by $[J^T]$ [39, 40]:

$$\left[J^T J\right]\left\{\Delta k^2\right\} = \left[J^T\right]\left\{E_m - E_c\right\} \qquad (7.4)$$

$[J^T J]$ is termed the Hessian matrix. The vector $\{\Delta k^2\}$, for which (7.4) is solved, is used to provide an update to $\{k_A^2\}$ at each iteration of a Gauss-Newton routine that converges to a least-squares estimate of the true property distribution $\{k_T^2\}$, that is [41],

$$\left\{k_A^2\right\}_{v+1} = \left\{k_A^2\right\}_v + \left\{\Delta k^2\right\}_v \qquad (7.5)$$

where v is the iteration number.

Two points should be made regarding (7.2). First, the forward solution $\{E_c\}$ must be accurate; the degree to which it approximates the actual fields at the O_E observation points determines the quality of the final image [42]. Second, in order to determine the elements of the Jacobian matrix $[J]$, some method must be found to determine the derivative of the electric field at each measurement site with respect to the property values at the L nodes of the parameter mesh. Both issues are addressed in the following section.

It should also be noted that the algorithm described in this section is applicable to both 2D and 3D problems, but the derivation in the following section is specific to two-dimensional scalar image reconstruction. In this case, transverse magnetic illumination is assumed, implying that the electric field is oriented in the z direction (out of the page) and can be treated as a scalar quantity [28].

Finally, the locations of the observation points and property-mesh nodes have deliberately been left arbitrary in order to facilitate later use of the dual mesh approach discussed in Chapter 2.

2.2   Hybrid Element Forward Solution

Solution of the Helmholtz equation (2.1), given some estimate $\{k_A^2\}$ of the property distribution—the "forward problem"—is required at each iteration of the method outlined above. In choosing a solution technique, certain conditions or goals have been kept in mind. (1) An optimal model-based imaging algorithm should capture its corresponding physical configuration as accurately as possible in numerical form [32]. (2) The computational size of the problem must be kept tractable, because not the forward problem must not only be solved, it must be solved at each iteration of the Newton's method inversion. N must therefore be minimized [43]. (3) Working against (2), spatial sampling of the electric field in the imaging zone (which must be calculated at all N nodes in order to determine $\{E_c\}$ in (7.4)) must be sufficiently dense to permit accurate field solution [44].

To satisfy these criteria, we have chosen a hybrid of the finite element (FE) and boundary element (BE) methods [45] for the two-dimensional problem. The FE method is well-suited for representing fields within a closed, heterogeneous, arbitrarily shaped imaging zone. The BE method, on the other hand, may be used to represent the homogeneous medium surrounding the imaging zone and may be coupled to the FE formulation by node sharing (Fig. 2) [46]. The region outside the FE zone, which contains all antennas, extends to infinity; however, given a medium sufficiently lossy to guarantee minimal reflections, only the surfaces of certain types of antennas and the interface of the BE and FE nodal systems need be discretized. The BE method entails a full-matrix problem (as opposed to the banded-matrix structure associated with FEs), so the number of shared boundary elements must be limited to prevent the problem from becoming computationally expensive.

The hybrid method provides a set of exact boundary conditions for the FE discretization [44, 47]. Furthermore, it allows the FE zone to be as small as possible by relegating large areas of homogenous space to treatment with the BE method. Keeping the FE zone small is helpful because the bandwidth of the matrices generated by the FE zone is proportional to the smallest cross-sectional dimension within the image field-of-view (and computational cost is proportional to the bandwidth squared) [42]. Wider nodal spacing over a fixed imaging field also reduces N, but an upper limit on internodal distance is determined by the need to accurately model the electric field across the imaging zone—in effect, by the operating frequency [43]. In practice, therefore, N can be reduced beyond a certain point only by minimizing the physical size of the FE mesh, which the hybrid method facilitates.

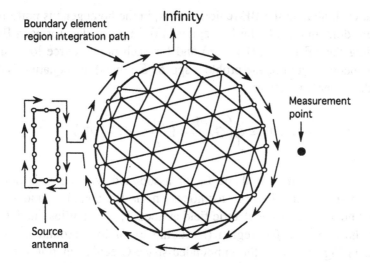

Figure 2. Schematic of hybrid method using both finite elements and boundary elements for solution of the forward problem. Filled triangle vertices are nodes in the FE mesh; open vertices are boundary element nodes shared with the FE mesh; open nodes on the source antenna are boundary element nodes not shared with the FE mesh.

Taking into account internal forcing functions and all nodes shared with the BE system, the FE region produces a matrix equation of the form $[A]\{E\} = [B]\{F\}$ or, more fully,

$$
\begin{bmatrix} A_{II} & A_{IB} \\ A_{BI} & A_{BB} \end{bmatrix} \begin{Bmatrix} E_I \\ E_B \end{Bmatrix} = \begin{bmatrix} 0 & 0 \\ 0 & B_{BB} \end{bmatrix} \begin{Bmatrix} 0 \\ F_B \end{Bmatrix} \tag{7.6}
$$

Here the subscripts I and B refer, respectively, to nodes interior to the FE mesh (I nodes) and to nodes shared by the FE and BE problems (B nodes): $I + B = N$. The dimensions of the four submatrices of $[A]$ are indicated by their subscripts; for example, submatrix A_{IB} is $I \times B$. Zeros indicate submatrices with all entries equal to zero. Similar notation is used for the column vectors $\{E\}$ and $\{F\}$, where $\{E\}$ is electric field and $\{F\} = \partial E / \partial n$; that is, E_I, E_B, and F_B are column vectors whose lengths are indicated by their respective subscripts.

Equation (7.6) comprises N equations in $I + 2B$ unknowns (i.e., the I unknowns of vector E_I, the B unknowns of vector E_B, and the B unknowns of vector F_B). Therefore, more equations are required for a solution. These are produced by applying Green's functions to the calculation of the electric field at each node in the BE region, that is, in the homogenous portion of the problem domain outside the FE region [45]. In particular, for each BE node bounding the FE mesh (B nodes) and for each point source located in the homogeneous region of the problem space (S points), an equation is derived from the Green's function:

$$\alpha_i E_i = \oint \left(G_i \frac{\partial E}{\partial n} - E \frac{\partial G_i}{\partial n} \right) ds + \langle f G_i \rangle \qquad (7.7)$$

Here α_i is a geometric shape factor associated with contour integration around a singularity (i.e., 0.5 for nodes on the BE boundary and 1.0 for all internal nodes); E_i is the electric field at node i; $\oint$ signifies line integration about the complete BE region (including excursions around antennas, as shown in Fig. 2); G_i is the unbounded-space Green's function for the two-dimensional Helmholtz equation (in this case, the Hankel function), singular at node i; $\partial E_i / \partial n = \nabla E_i \cdot \hat{n} = F$, the flux of the electric field across the line of integration at node i; $\partial G_i / \partial n = \nabla G_i \cdot \hat{n}$ is the flux of the Green's function across the line of integration at node i; f is a forcing function (e.g., a Dirac delta function) representing sources in the BE region; and $\langle \cdot \rangle$ indicates integration over the entire boundary of the BE region (i.e., from the FE mesh boundary out to infinity). Equation (7.7) is valid not only at nodes, but at *all* points within the BE region.

Application of (7.7) to all boundary and source nodes yields $B + S$ integral equations. The method of weighted residuals (see Ch. 2) is applied to these integral equations, using a Green's function centered at the mth node as the mth weighting function. This produces a set of linear equations that can be written

$$\begin{bmatrix} C_{BB} & C_{BS} \\ C_{SB} & C_{SS} \end{bmatrix} \begin{Bmatrix} F_B \\ F_S \end{Bmatrix} = \begin{bmatrix} D_{BB} & D_{BS} \\ D_{SB} & D_{SS} \end{bmatrix} \begin{Bmatrix} E_B \\ E_S \end{Bmatrix} + \begin{Bmatrix} Z_B \\ Z_S \end{Bmatrix} \qquad (7.8)$$

where the entries of [C] involve G_i, the entries of [D] involve α and $\partial G_i / \partial n$, the entries of {Z} include the $\langle f G_i \rangle$ terms from (7.7), and F_s and E_s are the flux and field associated with the discretization of the source antenna, one of which can be specified *a priori* while the other must be computed along with the other unknowns in the system.

Equations (7.6) and (7.8) can be solved simultaneously either by multiplying both sides of (7.6) by $[A]^{-1}$ and substituting for E_B in (7.8) or by multiplying both sides of (7.8) by $[C]^{-1}$ and substituting for F_B in (7.6). A complete forward solution (including a new $[A]$) must be computed at each iteration of the inverse solution, but because the electrical properties of the BE zone do not vary, $[C]^{-1}$ can be precalculated and stored in memory. For the breast-imaging application discussed in the next chapter, the latter approach is optimal.

After multiplying both sides of (7.8) by $[C]^{-1}$, we have

$$
\begin{Bmatrix} F_B \\ F_S \end{Bmatrix} = \begin{bmatrix} G_{BB} & G_{BS} \\ G_{SB} & G_{SS} \end{bmatrix} \begin{Bmatrix} E_B \\ E_S \end{Bmatrix} + \begin{bmatrix} CI_{BB} & CI_{BS} \\ CI_{SB} & CI_{SS} \end{bmatrix} \begin{Bmatrix} Z_B \\ Z_S \end{Bmatrix} \tag{7.9}
$$

where the sizes of the submatrices of $[G] = [C]^{-1}[D]$ and $[CI] = [C]^{-1}$ have been indicated by subscripts. Inserting the $\{F_B\}$ portion of (7.9) into (7.6) and rearranging produces

$$
\begin{bmatrix} A_{II} & A_{IB} \\ A_{BI} & A_{BB} - B_{BB}G_{BB} \end{bmatrix} \begin{Bmatrix} E_I \\ E_B \end{Bmatrix} = \begin{bmatrix} 0 & 0 \\ 0 & B_{BB}G_{BS} \end{bmatrix} \begin{Bmatrix} 0 \\ E_S \end{Bmatrix}
$$
$$
+ \begin{bmatrix} 0 & 0 \\ 0 & B_{BB}[CI_{BB} \ C_{BS}] \end{bmatrix} \begin{Bmatrix} 0 \\ Z_B \\ Z_S \end{Bmatrix} \tag{7.10}
$$

All subvectors on the right-hand side of (7.10) originate from antennas in the BE region and are therefore known. (Our treatment of (7.9) has assumed that E_S is known and that F_S is solved as part of the overall system. The methodology is sufficiently general to permit the use of antennas where F_S is known and E_S floats.)

Equation (7.10) is solved for E_I and E_B. The latter is substituted into (7.9) to compute F_B and F_S. The electric field at any point in the BE region (i.e., outside the FE region) can then be computed using equation (7.7).

A basic feature of this method is that terms coupled into the FE system from the BE equations are never more than B entries long. In practice, therefore, the computational impact on the FE problem of even large, complex structures outside the FE zone depends only on B, the number of nodes shared by the FE and BE systems [30].

2.3   Hybrid Element Reconstruction

Once the forward solution has been derived, the only term required to compute $\{\Delta k^2\}$ using (7.4) is the Jacobian matrix, [J]. For this, we need the derivatives of the electric field at all observation points with respect to the electrical property value k_j^2 at each node in the reconstruction parameter mesh. (As discussed further below, the parameter mesh is not necessarily the same as the mesh used to compute the electric field.) We begin by differentiating (7.6) and (7.8) with respect to k_j^2 and obtain (after rearrangement)

$$
\begin{bmatrix} \dfrac{\partial A_{II}}{\partial k_j^2} & \dfrac{\partial A_{IB}}{\partial k_j^2} \\[2mm] \dfrac{\partial A_{BI}}{\partial k_j^2} & \dfrac{\partial A_{BB}}{\partial k_j^2} \end{bmatrix} \begin{Bmatrix} E_I \\[2mm] E_B \end{Bmatrix} = - \begin{bmatrix} A_{II} & A_{IB} \\[2mm] A_{BI} & A_{BB} \end{bmatrix} \begin{Bmatrix} \dfrac{\partial E_I}{\partial k_j^2} \\[2mm] \dfrac{\partial E_B}{\partial k_j^2} \end{Bmatrix} + \begin{bmatrix} 0 & 0 \\[2mm] 0 & B_{BB} \end{bmatrix} \begin{Bmatrix} 0 \\[2mm] \dfrac{\partial F_B}{\partial k_j^2} \end{Bmatrix} \quad (7.11)
$$

$$
\text{and} \quad \begin{Bmatrix} \dfrac{\partial F_B}{\partial k_j^2} \\[4mm] \dfrac{\partial F_S}{\partial k_j^2} \end{Bmatrix} = \begin{bmatrix} G_{BB} \\[4mm] G_{SB} \end{bmatrix} \begin{Bmatrix} \dfrac{\partial E_B}{\partial k_j^2} \\[4mm] 0 \end{Bmatrix} \quad (7.12)
$$

In differentiating (7.6) to form (7.11) the chain rule has been applied, while in differentiating (7.8) to form (7.12) the derivatives of E_S, Z_B, and Z_S with respect to k_j^2 are all zero. E_I and E_B are obtained by solving (7.10), leaving $\partial E_I/\partial k_j^2$, $\partial E_B/\partial k_j^2$, and $\partial F_B/\partial k_j^2$ as unknowns in (7.11). However, $\partial F_B/\partial k_j^2$ is known in terms of $\partial E_B/\partial k_j^2$ from (7.12). Substituting (7.12) into (7.11) produces, after rearrangement,

$$
\begin{bmatrix} A_{II} & A_{IB} \\[4mm] A_{BI} & A_{BB} - B_{BB}G_{BB} \end{bmatrix} \begin{Bmatrix} \dfrac{\partial E_I}{\partial k_j^2} \\[4mm] \dfrac{\partial E_B}{\partial k_j^2} \end{Bmatrix} = - \begin{bmatrix} \dfrac{\partial A_{II}}{\partial k_j^2} & \dfrac{\partial A_{IB}}{\partial k_j^2} \\[4mm] \dfrac{\partial A_{BI}}{\partial k_j^2} & \dfrac{\partial A_{BB}}{\partial k_j^2} \end{bmatrix} \begin{Bmatrix} E_I \\[4mm] E_B \end{Bmatrix} \quad (7.13)
$$

The matrix on the left-hand side of this equation is the same as that used in the forward solution (7.10). Thus, the only terms required to solve (7.13) for $\partial E_I/\partial k_j^2$ and $\partial E_B/\partial k_j^2$ are the elements of matrix $\partial A/\partial k_j^2$. This necessitates examination of the terms in [A] as specified by the dual mesh analysis outlined in Chapter 2.

A measurement site may be modeled as one or more BE nodes (in which case the boundary of integration must make an excursion around that node or nodes) or as an arbitrary point in the BE region. The latter method shrinks the matrix problem but entails additional calculations. That is, when the observation site is an arbitrary point in the BE region, $\partial E/\partial k_j^2$ at that location must still be computed in order to construct the Jacobian matrix (see (7.2)). To do this we first compute $\partial F_B/\partial k_j^2$ and $\partial F_S/\partial k_j^2$ using (7.12). Once these vectors are known, (7.7) can be used to compute $\partial E/\partial k_j^2$ at the measurement site by differentiating both sides with respect to k_j^2 (which changes E to $\partial E/\partial k_j^2$ and $\partial E/\partial n$ to $\partial(\partial E/\partial k_j^2)/\partial n$) and solving for $\partial E/\partial k_j^2$ at the point within the BE region.

2   ANTENNA SELECTION

Any antenna to be employed in our system must be suitable for immersion in a liquid medium that (a) surrounds the target, (b) has electrical properties that are similar to those of the target, and (c) is lossy enough to permit the assumption that all fields propagate to infinity without reflection. (Alternative models have been proposed that incorporate perfectly reflecting or matched boundaries, but it is unclear how well either of these concepts will perform in practice.)

Antenna selection must accommodate both limitations in the numerical model and practical feasibility. Our earliest work [26] used liquid-filled waveguide radiators, which proved amenable to modeling and useful for actual imaging. They were relatively efficient and operated over a nominal bandwidth typical of waveguide aperture antennas, but were bulky. Given the lossiness of the medium, which limited the distance at which antennas could be positioned from the target, this bulkiness limited the number of antennas that could be placed around the target. Subsequently, we adopted simple monopole antennas, realizing quantifiable benefits [32]. This may seem counterintuitive, given the fact waveguides provide a more directed beam and therefore higher signal strength at the receiver antennas. However, a key element of any model-based approach is accurate matching to the physical system [41]. And while a waveguide antenna can be represented well by our mixed-element method, a monopole antenna allows even greater modeling accuracy for less effort. Further, the benefits of waveguide directionality were minimized by its radiation pattern, which was significantly broadened in practice by the lossy coupling medium.

Conventional wisdom suggests that monopole antennas are undesirable because they have a narrow operating bandwidth and cause surface currents that can propagate into the system hardware [48]. They are, nevertheless, well-suited to this imaging application. Figure 3 shows a monopole antenna's return loss in deionized water versus that in 0.9% saline. Note that the rapidly varying ripples in the deionized-water plot disappear in the saline results, an indication that spurious surface currents have been attenuated. Further, the antenna in saline has 10 dB or better return loss over the 100 to 1100 MHz bandwidth. While this return loss is not impressive by radar standards, it suffices for this transmission-mode measurement system—and the broad bandwidth is impressive. Broad bandwidth is essential for the log-magnitude/phase algorithm described below.

Finally, the simple structure of the monopole antenna allows compensation for nonactive antenna effects, as discussed in the next section.

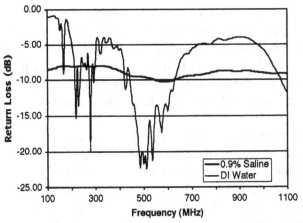

Figure 3. Return loss of monopole antenna for immersion in deionized (DI) water versus 0.9% saline solution. Lower return loss indicates better impedance match between the antenna and the liquid medium in which it is immersed.

3   NONACTIVE ANTENNA COMPENSATION

Simple one-transmitter, one-receiver arrangements are ideal for laboratory experiments because wave interactions with adjacent antennas do not occur and there is plenty of time to rotate the antennas and take more data. In a clinical system, however, examination time must be minimized. An antenna array is therefore logical because it enables the transmission and measurement to be switched electronically. Array utilization implies that the characteristics of the nonactive antennas must be incorporated into the forward model. Each nonactive antenna may, for example, be modeled as a perfect conductor [49], which is appealing because the resulting boundary conditions can be easily and accurately implemented in the numerical model in order to couple the signals to the metal structure for reradiation into the medium [50]. However, this approach ignores the fact that the nonactive antennas (like those actively transmitting and receiving) are connected to a cascade of microwave components that influences the reradiation. In practice, an incident signal couples to the antenna, propagates into the componentry path, and interacts with various impedance mismatches before it is reflected and reradiated [34].

To account for these interactions between the incident signal and the nonactive antennas, we have modified the microwave componentry attached to each antenna to present a matched termination during system operation when the antenna is nonactive (neither transmitting nor being used to make a measurement). Coupled energy is absorbed by the terminated antenna with minimal reradiation. This provides, in essence, the equivalent of first-order radiation boundary conditions at the surface of the nonactive antenna [51]. Furthermore, it eliminates mutual coupling between antenna elements. In mutual coupling, signals from a transmitting antenna couple to adjacent antennas, reradiate, and are coupled back to the transmitter with sufficient power to perturb its characteristic behavior. With matched terminations and a lossy medium, however, any signal reflected back to the original transmitter is too weak to have more than a modest impact [34].

Even so, the ring of antennas does perturb the overall field and can degrade image quality. Furthermore, the perturbation cannot be eliminated by subtracting a fixed contribution due to each nonactive antenna from each measured electric field value, because the impact of the nonactive antennas on a measurement is not a linear effect; the nonactive antennas must be fully represented as part of the complete forward solution [33]. (In the presentation that follows, compensation for nonactive antennas is discussed only with regard to the forward problem. Because the matrices of the inverse problem are similar, translation of these results to the inverse formulation [33, 34] is not given here.)

Figure 4 shows a schematic of the BE and FE regions, including a transmit antenna, a receive antenna, a nonactive antenna, and the BE integration path. Figure 4 is identical to Figure 2 except that the general source antenna, previously incorporated into the BE boundary integral, has been replaced by a point source. A single BE node is associated with each nonactive antenna (assumed to have radius R_A) and is located at its center.

In using (7.9) to eliminate F_B from (7.6), we assumed a fixed Dirichlet boundary condition (i.e., constant E_s) and allowed the flux $F_s = \partial E_s / \partial n$ at the antenna's surface to be determined as part of the overall solution. However, it would have been possible to assume, alternatively, a Neumann boundary condition—constant F_s—and allow the electric field E_s at the antenna surface to evolve. For the electromagnetic model applied to the

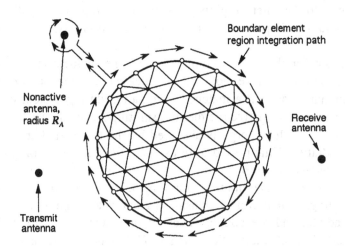

Figure 4. FE and BE systems for hybrid electric-field forward solution. Shown are a point illumination source and a single nonactive antenna of radius R_A (readily generalizable to multiple nonactive antennas). As in Fig. 2, FE nodes are filled vertices and BE nodes are open. A BE node (not shown) is located at the center of the nonactive antenna.

nonactive antennas, we assume a first-order radiation boundary condition on the circular antenna surface [50]:

$$E_i = -j\gamma \frac{\partial E_i}{\partial n} \tag{7.14}$$

Here γ is the effective impedance factor, $j = \sqrt{-1}$, E_i is the electric field at the ith BE node, and $\partial E_i / \partial n$ (i.e., F_i) is the electric field flux across the BE integration path at the ith node. Substituting (7.14) into (7.8) and rearranging produces

$$\begin{bmatrix} C_{BB} & C_{BS}+j\gamma D_{BS} \\ C_{SB} & C_{SS}+j\gamma D_{SS} \end{bmatrix} \begin{Bmatrix} F_B \\ F_S \end{Bmatrix} = \begin{bmatrix} D_{BB} & 0 \\ D_{SB} & 0 \end{bmatrix} \begin{Bmatrix} E_B \\ 0 \end{Bmatrix} + \begin{Bmatrix} Z_B \\ Z_S \end{Bmatrix} \tag{7.15}$$

F_B can now be computed as in Section 2.2, the difference being that [C] and [D] are altered by the addition of the nonactive antenna contour as described below.

We assume that R_A is sufficiently small so that the electric field can be treated as constant over the antenna surface. This allows us to model the antenna with a single BE node placed at its center, which significantly reduces the size of [C] and [D] (i.e., by keeping S, the number of source nodes, small). Values of γ and R_A can be determined empirically by first measuring the electric fields at the receiver sites both with and without the nonactive antennas present, producing a measured field perturbation. A computed version of the same experiment can be performed repeatedly, adjusting the empirically determined values of γ and R_A until the computed and measured field perturbations converge [52].

Addition of the nonactive antenna contour to the BE integration path (i.e., the path along which the contour integral of (7.7) is evaluated, yielding the entries of [C] and [D]) alters the matrix elements in (7.15) differently under two conditions: (1) the singularity of the Green's function G_i is coincident with the BE node at the center of a nonactive antenna, and (2) the singularity is located at another BE node (Fig. 5).

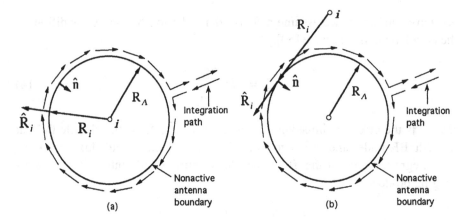

Figure 5. Two types of integration in nonactive antenna compensation. (a) Green's function singularity is positioned at BE node *i* at the center of the nonactive antenna; (b) singularity is located at BE node *i* outside a nonactive antenna. (Figure not drawn to scale.)

When the Green's-function singularity is positioned at the center of the nonactive antenna (Fig. 5a), the integrations are straightforward: the distance argument is measured from the center of the nonactive antenna to the integration path along the imaging region boundary. The first term on the right-hand side of (7.7) then produces

$$\oint_{antenna} \left(\frac{\partial E}{\partial n} G_i - E \frac{\partial G_i}{\partial n} \right) ds \approx \frac{\partial E_i}{\partial n} G_i \int_0^{2\pi} R_A \, d\theta - \frac{\partial G_i}{\partial n} E_i \int_0^{2\pi} R_A \, d\theta \qquad (7.16)$$

for the portion of the contour integral that passes around the nonactive antenna modeled by BE node *i*, where θ is the integration angle about the center of the antenna, R_A is assumed to be sufficiently small that E (and, therefore, $\partial E/\partial n$) is constant along the integration path. Also, use has been made of the fact G_i and $\partial G_i/\partial n$ are constant at a fixed distance from the singularity at the antenna center and are therefore not functions of θ. Since both integrals with respect to θ evaluate to $2\pi R_A$, the right-hand side of (7.16) can be rewritten

$$2\pi R_A \left[\frac{\partial E_i}{\partial n} G_i(R_A) + \frac{\partial G_i(R_A)}{\partial R} E_i \right] \qquad (7.17)$$

where evaluation of G_i at R_A has been emphasized. There are still two unknowns, E_i and $\partial E_i/\partial n$. We invoke the impedance relationship (7.14) to eliminate the former and obtain

$$2\pi R_A \frac{\partial E_i}{\partial n}\left[G_i(R_A) - j\gamma\frac{\partial G_i(R_A)}{\partial n}\right] \tag{7.18}$$

This term produces contributions to the diagonal of the [C] matrix in (7.15).

When the singularity in G_i is centered at a BE node on the boundary of the FE region or at the center of another nonactive antenna (Fig. 5b), then we again assume that E and $\partial E/\partial n$ are constant for the portion of the contour which encircles the nonactive antenna. The distance argument of the Green's function is not constant in this case but is a function of the angle from BE node i to each point on the contour. Denoting this distance by $R_i(\theta)$, we have

$$\oint_{antenna}\left(\frac{\partial E}{\partial n}G_i - \frac{\partial G_i}{\partial n}E\right)ds \approx R_A\frac{\partial E_A}{\partial n}\int_0^{2\pi} G_i(R_i(\theta))\,d\theta$$

$$- R_A E_A \int_0^{2\pi} \frac{\partial G_i(R_i(\theta))}{\partial R}\hat{\mathbf{R}}_i(\theta)\cdot\hat{\mathbf{n}}(\theta)\,d\theta$$

$$\approx R_A\frac{\partial E_A}{\partial n}\left[\int_0^{2\pi} G_i(R_i(\theta))\,d\theta + j\gamma\int_0^{2\pi}\frac{\partial G_i(R_i(\theta))}{\partial R}\hat{\mathbf{R}}_i(\theta)\cdot\hat{\mathbf{n}}(\theta)\,d\theta\right] \tag{7.19}$$

where E_A and $\partial E_A/\partial n$ are the electric field and flux on the antenna surface, respectively (and are related to each other through (7.14)), and R_i, $\hat{\mathbf{R}}_i$, and $\hat{\mathbf{n}}$ are written as functions of θ to stress their angular dependence. The right-hand side of (7.19) is easily integrated by Gaussian quadrature or can be further approximated as

$$2\pi R_A G_i(R_i)\frac{\partial E_A}{\partial n} \tag{7.20}$$

when the distance from the singularity to the nonactive antenna is large compared to R_A (i.e., $R_i \gg R_A$ and can be considered a constant), since in this case

$$\int_0^{2\pi} \hat{\mathbf{R}}_i(\theta) \cdot \hat{\mathbf{n}}(\theta) d\theta \to 0 \qquad (7.21)$$

The approximation given in (7.20) is valid when the BE node on which the Green's function is centered is distant from the antenna in question. With $F = \partial E/\partial n$ at the nonactive antenna site given by (7.20), we can find E at that point through (7.14).

Equation (7.20) and evaluation of (7.19) produce contributions to [C] in (7.15) in the column associated with the BE node at the center of one monopole antenna.

4   LOG-MAGNITUDE, UNWRAPPED-PHASE RECONSTRUCTION ALGORITHM

When the target is electrically high-contrast with respect to the background medium, phase differences in excess of π radians may occur between observation points. In complex-plane representation [26, 27, 53, 54], electric-field values are, by default, mapped into the Riemann sheet bounded by $-\pi$ and $+\pi$ through the addition or subtraction of multiples of 2π. That is, antenna-to-antenna phase variations that are actually smooth may appear grossly discontinuous when they pass over $+\pi$ and suddenly reappear at $-\pi$ in the recorded data. Under these conditions, image reconstruction may fail due to the nonunique nature of the gradient in (7.4) (i.e., $[J^\tau]\{E_m - E_c\}$) without reliance on a priori information about the size and structure of the target, antenna placement, and the inherent smoothness of phase variation,.

To cope with large phase, we have devised an alternate formulation of the general inverse algorithm based on expanding the log-magnitude and unwrapped phase components of the electric fields in a truncated Taylor series about an approximate solution [16]. While the formulation necessitates phase unwrapping of the measured and computed data, it has two major benefits. The first is a reduced dependence on a priori information, and the second is a correction in the weighting of field values measured by receiver antennas opposite the transmitter relative to more peripheral ones. This bias is mainly due to attenuation of signals propagating through the medium compared to measurements on the sides closer to the transmitter, where values may be orders of magnitude greater.

In practice, peripheral measurements are influenced primarily by property contrast between the overall (large) object and background, while signals propagating through the object contain significantly more information about structures within. Our algorithm, which we call log-magnitude/phase form (LMPF) reconstruction, emphasizes the relative differences between the measured and computed fields for both log magnitude and phase. Further-more, it utilizes field values and (for the Jacobian matrix) derivatives already computed, thus adding minimal computational cost (relative to its complex-form counterpart).

Below, we derive the $\{\Delta k^2\}$ update computation in the LMPF algorithm that is analogous to (7.4) in the conventional approach. We then describe strategies for unwrapping the phase terms for the measured and computed field terms and discuss issues complicating its use.

4.1   LMPF Reconstruction

As in the complex-form approach, the electric-field values are computed at the points of measurement at each iteration in the LMPF scheme. However, it is necessary to separate the log of the electric-field magnitude ($\Gamma = \log(E_{mag})$) from the electric-field phase Φ. It is also useful to separate k^2 into its real and imaginary components, k_{Re}^2 and k_{Im}^2. The true log elec-tric-field magnitude and electric field phase vectors, Γ_T and Φ_T, which are functions of the true electrical property distribution (having real and imagi-nary parts $_T k_{Re}^2$ and $_T k_{Im}^2$), are each approximated as a three-term Taylor se-ries expanded around an approximate electrical property profile represented by the L-dimensional vectors $_A k_{Re}^2$ and $_A k_{Im}^2$, i.e.,

$$\Gamma_T\left(_T k_{Re}^2,\ _T k_{Im}^2\right) \approx \Gamma_A\left(_A k_{Re}^2,\ _A k_{Im}^2\right) + \left.\frac{\partial \Gamma_A}{\partial k_{Re}^2}\right|_A \Delta k_{Re}^2 + \left.\frac{\partial \Gamma_A}{\partial k_{Im}^2}\right|_A \Delta k_{Im}^2 \quad (7.22)$$

and

$$\Phi_T\left(_T k_{Re}^2,\ _T k_{Im}^2\right) \approx \Phi_A\left(_A k_{Re}^2,\ _A k_{Im}^2\right) + \left.\frac{\partial \Phi_A}{\partial k_{Re}^2}\right|_A \Delta k_{Re}^2 + \left.\frac{\partial \Phi_A}{\partial k_{Im}^2}\right|_A \Delta k_{Im}^2 \quad (7.23)$$

where $\partial\Gamma_A/\partial k_{Re}^2$, $\partial\Gamma_A/\partial k_{Im}^2$, $\partial\Phi_A/\partial k_{Re}^2$, and $\partial\Phi_A/\partial k_{Im}^2$ are $O_{IM} \times L$ matrices; $\Delta k_{Re}^2 = {}_T k_{Re}^2 - {}_A k_{Re}^2$; and $\Delta k_{Im}^2 = {}_T k_{Im}^2 - {}_A k_{Im}^2$.

Much as in (7.1) and (7.2), this process can be written as

$$\left[\quad J \quad\right]\left\{\begin{array}{c}\Delta k_{Re}^2 \\ \Delta k_{Im}^2\end{array}\right\} = \left\{\begin{array}{c}\Gamma_m - \Gamma_c \\ \Phi_m - \Phi_c\end{array}\right\} \quad (7.24)$$

where [J] is the $2O_{IM} \times 2L$ Jacobian matrix and Γ_m, Γ_c, Φ_m, and Φ_c are the measured and calculated log-magnitude and phase vectors (all length O_{IM}). This set of equations can also be solved as a least-squares problem using the method of normal equations. We multiply both sides of (7.24) by $[J^T]$ to obtain [39]

$$\left[\; J^TJ \; \right] \left\{ \begin{array}{c} \Delta k_{Re}^2 \\ \Delta k_{Im}^2 \end{array} \right\} = \left[\; J^T \; \right] \left\{ \begin{array}{c} \Gamma_m - \Gamma_c \\ \Phi_m - \Phi_c \end{array} \right\} \tag{7.25}$$

where $[J^TJ]$ is the $2O_{IM} \times 2L$ Hessian matrix. The Jacobian matrix is

$$\left[\begin{array}{cc} \dfrac{\partial \Gamma}{\partial k_{Re}^2} & \dfrac{\partial \Gamma}{\partial k_{Im}^2} \\[3mm] \dfrac{\partial \Phi}{\partial k_{Re}^2} & \dfrac{\partial \Phi}{\partial k_{Im}^2} \end{array} \right] \tag{7.26}$$

where each submatrix is $O_{IM} \times L$. The elements of the four submatrices in (7.26) can be written

$$\left(\frac{\partial \Gamma}{\partial k_{Re}^2} \right)_{j,\ell} = \frac{1}{|E|_j^2} \left((E_{Re})_j \frac{\partial (E_{Re})_j}{\partial (k_{Re}^2)_\ell} + (E_{Im})_j \frac{\partial (E_{Im})_j}{\partial (k_{Re}^2)_\ell} \right)$$

$$\left(\frac{\partial \Gamma}{\partial k_{Im}^2} \right)_{j,\ell} = \frac{1}{|E|_j^2} \left((E_{Re})_j \frac{\partial (E_{Re})_j}{\partial (k_{Im}^2)_\ell} + (E_{Im})_j \frac{\partial (E_{Im})_j}{\partial (k_{Im}^2)_\ell} \right)$$

$$\left(\frac{\partial \Phi}{\partial k_{Re}^2} \right)_{j,\ell} = \frac{1}{|E|_j^2} \left((E_{Im})_j \frac{\partial (E_{Re})_j}{\partial (k_{Re}^2)_\ell} - (E_{Re})_j \frac{\partial (E_{Im})_j}{\partial (k_{Re}^2)_\ell} \right) \tag{7.27}$$

$$\left(\frac{\partial \Phi}{\partial k_{Im}^2} \right)_{j,\ell} = \frac{1}{|E|_j^2} \left((E_{Im})_j \frac{\partial (E_{Re})_j}{\partial (k_{Im}^2)_\ell} - (E_{Re})_j \frac{\partial (E_{Im})_j}{\partial (k_{Im}^2)_\ell} \right)$$

where j ranges from 1 to O_{IM}; ℓ ranges from 1 to L; the log magnitude Γ and phase Φ are expressed in terms of the real and imaginary parts of the electric field, E_{Re} and E_{Im}; and

$$|E|_j^2 = \left(E_{Re}\right)_j^2 + \left(E_{Im}\right)_j^2 \tag{7.28}$$

To find the partial derivatives of $(E_{Re})_j$ and $(E_{Im})_j$ required in (7.27), we differentiate both sides of the matrix representation of the forward solution, $[A]\{E\} = \{b\}$ (still maintaining the previous complex representations), first with respect to $(k_{Re}^2)_u$ and second with respect to $(k_{Im}^2)_u$. This yields two equations,

$$\left\{\frac{\partial E}{\partial\left(k_{Re}^2\right)_u}\right\} = \left[\begin{array}{c} A \end{array}\right]^{-1} \left[\frac{\partial A}{\partial\left(k_{Re}^2\right)_u}\right]\{E\} \tag{7.29}$$

and

$$\left\{\frac{\partial E}{\partial\left(k_{Im}^2\right)_u}\right\} = \left[\begin{array}{c} A \end{array}\right]^{-1} \left[\frac{\partial A}{\partial\left(k_{Im}^2\right)_u}\right]\{E\} \tag{7.30}$$

The nonzero terms of $[A]$ are

$$\alpha_{j,u} = \left\langle -\nabla\phi_j \cdot \nabla\phi_u \right\rangle + \left\langle \phi_j \phi_u \sum_{\ell=1}^{L}\left[\left(k_{Re}^2\right)_\ell + i\left(k_{Im}^2\right)_\ell\right]\psi_\ell \right\rangle \tag{7.31}$$

where ϕ_j and ϕ_u are basis functions from the FE representation of the electric field and ψ_ℓ is a basis function from the FE representation of the material property distribution, i.e.,

$$k_{Re}^2(x,y) = \sum_{\ell=1}^{L}\left(k_{Re}^2\right)_\ell \psi_\ell(x,y) \quad \text{and} \quad k_{Im}^2(x,y) = \sum_{\ell=1}^{L}\left(k_{Im}^2\right)_\ell \psi_\ell(x,y) \tag{7.32}$$

The entries of matrix $\partial A/\partial(k_{Re}^2)_\ell$ in (7.29) are zero except when ψ_ℓ is nonzero, in which case $\partial\alpha_{\ell,j}/\partial(k_{Re}^2)_\ell = \langle\phi_u\phi_j\psi_\ell\rangle$. Likewise, all terms of $\partial A/\partial(k_{Im}^2)_\ell$ in (7.30) are zero except where ψ_ℓ is nonzero, in which case $\partial\alpha_{\ell,j}/\partial(k_{Im}^2)_\ell = i\langle\phi_u\phi_j\psi_\ell\rangle$.

From (7.29) and (7.30) we can extract the derivatives required to construct the Jacobian, (7.26), via substitution in (7.27) and the relationships

$$\frac{\partial E_j}{\partial\left(k_{Re}^2\right)_\ell} = \frac{\partial\left(E_{Re}\right)_j}{\partial\left(k_{Re}^2\right)_\ell} + i\frac{\partial\left(E_{Im}\right)_j}{\partial\left(k_{Re}^2\right)_\ell} \tag{7.33}$$

$$\text{and} \qquad \frac{\partial E_j}{\partial \left(k_{\text{Im}}^2\right)_\ell} = \frac{\partial \left(E_{\text{Re}}\right)_j}{\partial \left(k_{\text{Im}}^2\right)_\ell} + i \frac{\partial \left(E_{\text{Im}}\right)_j}{\partial \left(k_{\text{Im}}^2\right)_\ell} \qquad (7.34)$$

Additionally, because $\partial A/\partial(k_{\text{Re}}^2)_\ell$ and $\partial A/\partial(k_{\text{Im}}^2)_\ell$ in (7.29) and (7.30) differ only by a factor of i,

$$\frac{\partial \left(E_{\text{Re}}\right)_j}{\partial \left(k_{\text{Im}}^2\right)_\ell} = -\frac{\partial \left(E_{\text{Im}}\right)_j}{\partial \left(k_{\text{Re}}^2\right)_\ell} \quad \text{and} \quad \frac{\partial \left(E_{\text{Im}}\right)_j}{\partial \left(k_{\text{Im}}^2\right)_\ell} = -\frac{\partial \left(E_{\text{Re}}\right)_j}{\partial \left(k_{\text{Re}}^2\right)_\ell} \qquad (7.35)$$

This improves algorithmic efficiency because all four components in (7.27) can be computed with a single matrix back-substitution.

4.2   Phase Unwrapping

For relatively low frequencies and fine levels of electrical property mesh discretization, elements of the two lower submatrices of the Jacobian matrix in (7.26)—namely, $(\partial \Phi / \partial (k_{\text{Re}}^2))_{j,\ell}$ and $(\partial \Phi / \partial (k_{\text{Im}}^2))_{j,\ell}$—typically do not need to be unwrapped because phase changes at a measurement site due to perturbation of the electrical properties of a single node in the property mesh rarely exceed π. However, the measured and computed electric-field phases in (7.25), Φ_m and Φ_c, do require phase unwrapping.

We begin by evaluating the phase at all receiver sites for a given transmitter. Either the absolute phase or the relative phase with respect to a calibration common to both the measured and computed fields can be used.

For phase unwrapping of the computed field, Φ_c, provided by the forward solution at a given iteration of the imaging algorithm, we compare phase values at receiver sites counterclockwise around the target region, adding or subtracting 2π whenever the difference between adjacent sites exceeds π (i.e., whenever the antenna-to-antenna phase curve suffers a discontinuity due to wrapping of $\pi + x$ to $-\pi + x$). However, at high frequencies and when the receiver sites are separated by electrically large distances, nonartifactual interantenna phase differences greater than π are possible. This problem can be alleviated by computing additional electric-field values at positions intermediate between receiver sites and subsequently re-applying the phase unwrapping scheme. Unwrapping of the computed phase can thus be efficiently incorporated into our existing numerical algorithm.

Phase unwrapping is not as readily accomplished for the measured data, Φ_m. There is a physical lower limit to receiver antenna spacing, making it impossible to keep phase differences between adjacent antennas below a certain limit. As with the calculated phase, it is entirely possible to observe phase differences between adjacent receivers greater than π, especially at high frequencies. Receiver data does not provide electric field values at positions intermediate to receiver sites that can be used to distinguish phase differences greater and less than π (as calculated intermediate values are used in unwrapping Φ_c). To solve this problem, we take advantage of the broadband data available from our current data acquisition system. These data are a collection of imaging measurement sets for a given target, each gathered at a different frequency. When the interval between acquisition frequencies is sufficiently small, the scattered field values for a given transmitter/receiver pair will not vary significantly. The phase of the measured electric fields for each transmit/receive antenna pair is unwrapped by comparing phases of adjacent receiver antennas for the lowest-frequency data, for which phase shift is minimal; these values are then compared to those for each transmitter/receiver pair at a slightly higher frequency, yielding a highly probable value for the unwrapped phase at that frequency. This value can in turn be used to guide unwrapping at the next-highest frequency, and so on. When the operating frequency range is sampled at relatively close intervals, this process can be automated in a robust manner.

5   CONFORMAL MESH APPROACH

The microwave imaging approach is distinguished from the other tomographic modalities, EIS and NIR, by the fact that the antennas (sensors) do not directly contact the breast. The imaging zone can be any convex, continuous region surrounding the breast within the antenna array (usually a circular or elliptical region, given our circular antenna array). When the imaging zone is considerably larger than the breast, however, the image can become degraded because a significant fraction of the parameter-mesh nodes are needed to represent the property gradient between the breast and surrounding liquid. Given limited N, this inevitably reduces resolution within the breast itself.

We have developed a "conformal mesh" approach whereby the property mesh can be conformed to the actual breast perimeter [55]. The property distribution used in the forward solution can be set to a step function at the breast perimeter by utilizing the flexibility of the hybrid forward method, which couples a BE representation of the surrounding, electrically homogeneous medium with an FE description of the heterogeneous breast. If the breast contour can be determined exactly, the final image will not be degraded by oversampling of the boundary gradient. (The boundary gradient, because of the regularization applied during the reconstruction process, can extend well inside the physical breast boundary.) Our studies have demonstrated that even when the contour is not known exactly, image quality improves progressively as the conformal mesh perimeter approaches the exact breast boundary. This makes it worthwhile to approximate the boundary using a convenient regular shape (e.g., ellipse) that best fits the breast contour.

The challenge here is to determine the breast boundary. Suggested approaches have included (1) using an optical laser or ultrasound system to illuminate the breast from multiple angles to deduce its surface; (2) examining broadband projection data for phase and magnitude changes indicating the boundary; (3) recovering an image of the breast using a large, circular mesh concentric with the antenna array and then performing edge detection (automated or user-guided) on the image. The first method faces the difficulty of integrating extra hardware with the microwave array without disrupting the imaging signals, but could produce accurate measures of the contour. The latter two methods use data that have already been acquired. We have had some success with the third approach, using an image reconstructed on the large, antenna-concentric, default mesh as a guide for superimposing a finer, elliptical mesh with unchanged N on the area of interest (Fig. 6).

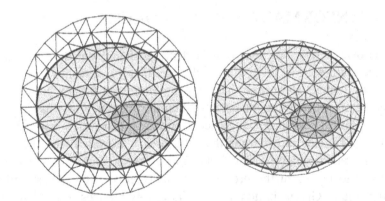

Figure 6. Conformal mesh method applied to a hypothetical elliptical target containing an anomaly. Sixteen fixed monopole antennas (not shown) encircle the region. *Left*: target with circular, antenna-concentric mesh. *Right*: Same target with elliptical, conformal mesh having the same number of nodes as the circular mesh.

REFERENCES

[1]   J. Overgaard et al., "Randomized trial of hyperthermia as adjuvant to radiotherapy for recurrent or metastatic malignant melanoma." *Lancet*, Vol. 345, 1995, pp. 540–543.

[2]   J. van der Zee et al., "Comparison of radiotherapy alone with radiotherapy plus hyperthermia in locally advanced pelvic tumours: A prospective, randomized, multicentre trial." *Lancet*, Vol. 355, 2000, pp. 1119–1125.

[3]   M. I. Skolnik, *Introduction to Radar Systems* (New York: McGraw-Hill, 1980).

[4]   S. Webb, *The Physics of Medical Imaging* (Philadelphia: Hilger, 1988).

[5]   *Mammography and Beyond: Developing Techniques for the Early Detection of Breast Cancer* (Washington, D.C.: Institute of Medicine, National Academy Press, 2000).

[6]   E. Schmid, "Is there reliable experimental evidence for a low-dose RBE of about 4 for mammography x-rays relative to 200 kV x-rays?" *Radiat. Res.*, Vol. 158, 2002, pp. 778–781.

[7]   C. Gabriel, S. Gabriel and E. Corthout, "The dielectric properties of biological tissues: I. Literature survey." *Phys. Med. Biol.*, Vol. 41, 1996, pp. 2231–2249.

[8]   S. Gabriel, R. W. Lau, and C. Gabriel, "The dielectric properties of biological tissues: II. Measurements on the frequency range 10 Hz to 20 GHz." *Phys. Med. Biol.*, Vol. 41, 1996, pp. 2251–2269.

[9]   S. Gabriel, R. W. Lau, and C. Gabriel. "The dielectric properties of biological tissues: III. Parametric models for the dielectric spectrum of tissues." *Phys. Med. Biol.*, Vol. 41, 1996, pp. 2271–2293.

[10]   K. R. Foster and H. P. Schwan, "Dielectric properties of tissues and biological materials: A critical review." *Crit. Rev. Biomed. Eng.*, Vol. 17, 1989, pp. 25–104.

[11]   R. F. Harringon, *Field Computation by Moment Methods* (Malabar, FL: Krieger, 1982).

[12]   K. R. Foster and J. L. Schepps, "Dielectric properties of tumor and normal tissues at radio through microwave frequencies." *J. Micro. Power*, Vol. 16, 1981, pp. 107–119.

[13]   L. E. Larson and J. H. Jacobi, *Medical Applications of Microwave Imaging* (New York: IEEE, 1986).

[14]   M. Slaney, A. C. Kak, and L. E. Larsen, "Limitations of imaging with first-order diffraction tomography." *IEEE Trans. Microwave Theory Tech.*, Vol. 32, 1984, pp. 860–874.

[15]   N. Joachimowicz, C. Pichot, and J. R. Hugonin, "Inverse scattering: An iterative numerical method for electromagnetic imaging." *IEEE Trans. Antennas Propagat.*, Vol. 39, 1991, pp. 1742–1752.

[16]   P. M. Meaney et al., "Microwave image reconstruction utilizing log-magnitude and unwrapped phase to improve high-contrast object recovery." *IEEE Trans. Med. Imag.*, Vol. 20, 2001, pp. 104–116.

[17]   E. J. Bond et al., "Microwave imaging via space-time beamforming for early detection of breast cancer." *IEEE Trans. Ant. Prop.*, Vol. 51, 2003, pp. 1690–1705.

[18]   S. C. Hagness, A. Taflove, and J. E. Bridges, "Two-dimensional FDTD analysis of a pulsed microwave confocal system for breast cancer detection: Fixed-focus and antenna-array sensors." *IEEE Trans. Biomed. Eng.*, Vol. 45, 1998, pp. 1470–479.

[19]   S. C. Hagness, A. Taflove, and J. E. Bridges, "Three-dimensional FDTD analysis of pulsed microwave confocal system for breast cancer detection: Design of an antenna-array element." *IEEE Trans. Antennas Propag.*, Vol. 47, 1999, pp. 783–791.

[20]   E. C. Fear and M. A. Stuchly, "Microwave detection of breast cancer." *IEEE Trans. Microw. Theory Tech.*, Vol. 48, 2000, pp. 1854–1863.

[21]   E. C. Fear et al., "Confocal microwave imaging for breast cancer detection: Localization of tumors in three dimensions." *IEEE Trans. Biomed. Eng.*, Vol. 49, 2002, pp. 812–822.

[22]   E. C. Fear et al., "Enhancing breast tumor detection with near-field imaging." *IEEE Microwave Magazine*, Vol. 3, 2002, pp. 48–56.

[23] K. L. Carr et al., "Radiometric sensing: an adjuvant to mammography to determine breast biopsy." *IEEE International Microwave Symposium*, Boston, MA, 2000, pp. 929–932.

[24] S. Mouty et al., "Microwave radiometric imaging for the characterisation of breast tumors." *European Physical Journal: Applied Physics*, Vol. 10, 2000, pp. 73–78.

[25] R. A. Kruger et al., "Thermoacoustic computed tomography of the breast at 434 MHz." *IEEE MTT-S International Microwave Symposium Digest*, 1999, pp. 591–594.

[26] A. E. Bulyshev et al., "Computational modeling of three-dimensional microwave tomography of breast cancer." *IEEE Trans. Biomed. Eng.*, Vol. 48, 2001, pp. 1053–1056.

[27] Z. Q. Zhang et al., "Microwave breast imaging: 3-D forward scattering simulation." *IEEE Trans. Biomed. Eng.*, Vol. 50, 2003, pp. 1180–1189.

[28] P. M. Meaney, K. D. Paulsen, and T. P. Ryan, "Two-dimensional hybrid element image reconstruction for TM illumination." *IEEE Trans. Ant. Prop.*, Vol. 43, 1995, pp. 239–247.

[29] N. Joachimowicz, C. Pichot, and J. R. Hugonin, "Inverse scattering: An iterative numerical method for electromagnetic imaging." *IEEE Trans. Antennas Prop.*, Vol. 39, 1991, pp. 1742–1752.

[30] S. Caorsi, G. G. Gragnani, and M. Pastorino, "A multi-view microwave imaging system for two-dimensional penetrable objects." *IEEE Trans. Microwave Theory Tech.*, Vol. 39, 1991, pp. 845–851.

[31] K. D. Paulsen and D. R. Lynch, "Calculation of interior values by the boundary element method." *Commun. Appl. Numerical Methods*, Vol. 5, 1989, pp. 7–14.

[32] D. H. Schaubert and P. M. Meaney, "Efficient calculation of scattering by inhomogeneous dielectric bodies." *IEEE Trans. Antennas Prop.*, Vol. 34, 1986.

[33] P. M. Meaney, K. D. Paulsen, and J. T. Chang, "Near-field microwave imaging of biologically based materials using a monopole transceiver system." *IEEE Trans. Microwave Theory Tech.*, Vol. 46, 1998, pp. 31–45.

[34] K. D. Paulsen and P. M. Meaney, "Compensation for nonactive array element effects in a microwave imaging system: Part I—forward solution vs. measured data comparison." *IEEE Trans. Med. Imag.*, Vol. 18, 1999, pp. 508–518.

[35] P. M. Meaney et al., "Compensation for nonactive array element effects in a microwave imaging system: Part II—imaging results." *IEEE Trans. Med. Imag.*, Vol. 18, 1999, pp. 508–518.

[36] D. Li, P. M. Meaney, and K. D. Paulsen, "Conformal microwave imaging for breast cancer detection." *IEEE Trans. Microwave Theory Tech.*, Vol. 51, 2003, 1779–1186.

[37] K. D. Paulsen et al., "A dual mesh scheme for finite element based reconstruction algorithms." *IEEE Trans. Med. Imag.*, Vol. 14, 1995, pp. 504–514.

[38] P. M. Meaney et al., "A two-stage microwave image reconstruction procedure for inverse internal feature extraction." *Med. Phys.*, Vol. 28, 2001, pp. 2358–2369.

[39] G. Demoment, "Image reconstruction and restoration: Overview of common estimation structures and problems." *IEEE Trans. Acoust., Speech, Signal Processing*, Vol. 37, 1989, pp. 2024–2036.

[40] G. H. Golub and C. F. van Loan, *Matrix Computations*, 2nd ed. (Baltimore, MD: Johns Hopkins Univ. Press, 1989).

[41] B. Kaltenbacher, "Newton-type methods for ill-posed problems." *Inverse Probl.*, Vol. 13, 1997, pp. 729–753.

[42] E. Demidenko, "Asymptotic properties of nonlinear mixed effects models," in *Modeling Longitudinal and Spatially Correlated Data* (New York: Springer-Verlag, 1997), pp. 47–62.

[43] K. D. Paulsen and W. Liu, "Memory and operations count scaling for coupled finite element and boundary element systems of equations." *Int. J. Numerical Methods in Eng.*, Vol. 33, 1992, pp. 1289–1304.

[44] K. D. Paulsen, D. R. Lynch, and J. W. Strohbehn, "Three-dimensional finite, boundary, and hybrid element solutions of the Maxwell equations for lossy dielectric media." *IEEE Trans. Microwave Theory Tech.*, Vol. MTT-36, 1988, pp. 682–693.

[45] D. R. Lynch. K. D. Paulsen, and J. W. Strohbehn, "Hybrid element method for unbounded electromagnetic problems in hyperthermia." *Int. J. Numer. Methods Eng.*, Vol. 23, 1986, pp. 1915–1937.

[46] K. Yashiro and S. Ohkawa, "Boundary element method for electromagnetic scattering from cylinders." *IEEE Trans. Antennas Prop.*, Vol. 33, 1985, pp. 383–389.

[47] M. Johnsen, K. D. Paulsen, and F. E. Werner, "Radiation boundary conditions for finite element solutions of generalized wave equations." *Int. J. Numer. Meth. Fluids*, Vol. 12, 1991, pp. 765–783.

[48] P. M. Meaney et al., "An active microwave imaging system for reconstruction of 2-D electrical property distributions." *IEEE Trans. Biomed. Eng.*, Vol. 42, 1995, pp. 1017–1026.

[49] D. Franza, N. Joachimowicz, and J. C. Boloney, "SICS: A sensor interaction compensation scheme for microwave imaging," *IEEE Trans. Antennas Prop.*, Vol. 50, 2002, pp. 211–216.

[50] C. A. Balanis, *Antenna Theory: Analysis and Design* (New York: Harper & Row, 1982), pp. 62–67.

[51] T. B. A. Senior and J. L. Volakis, *Approximate Boundary Conditions in Electromagnetics* (London: Institute of Electrical Engineers, 1995).

[52] G. F. F. Seber and C. J. Wild, *Nonlinear Regression* (New York: Wiley, 1989).

[53] S. Caorsi, G. L. Gragnani, and M. Pastorino, "Reconstruction of dielectric permittivity distributions in arbitrary 2-D inhomogeneous biological bodies by a multiview microwave numerical method." *IEEE Trans. Med. Imag.*, Vol. 12, 1993, pp. 232–239.

[54] Q. H. Liu et al., "Active microwave imaging 1-2 D forward and inverse scattering methods." *IEEE Trans. Microwave Theory Tech.*, Vol. 50, 2002, pp. 123–133.

[55] D. Li, P. M. Meaney, K. D. Paulsen, "Conformal microwave imaging for breast cancer techniques." *IEEE Trans. Microwave Theory Tech.*, Vol. 51, 2003, pp. 1179–1186.

Chapter 8

MICROWAVE IMAGING: HARDWARE AND RESULTS

Paul M. Meaney, Ph.D. and Dun Li, Ph.D.

1   INTRODUCTION

Simulations are useful for assessing early-stage design options and for aiding in the understanding of unexpected experimental behavior. However, experimenting with a clinical prototype is essential for illuminating practical issues, many of which are difficult to simulate (e.g., depth of submersion of the antenna array in the coupling medium), and allows assessment of image quality under conditions similar to those that occur during actual patient exams. Ultimately, using a prototype with patients is the only way to verify certain performance characteristics, such as whether the coupling medium will work appropriately, whether the system is comfortable for women, whether exam duration is tolerable, and so on. Results from such testing informed changes integrated into our second-generation prototype, and will continue to be important during system development.

Our hardware design process has been structured around four basic themes: simplicity, modularity, spectral capability, and reliability [1].

Simplicity. Our image-reconstruction algorithm uses a model-based Gauss-Newton iterative approach. It is, therefore, imperative that our numerical model accurately represent the physical interactions occurring in the illumination chamber. Use of a lossy coupling medium (fluid bath) to minimize out-of-plane and tank-wall reflections, along with monopole antennas that can be represented as simple line sources, makes accurate modeling feasible while keeping the hardware design simple and flexible. In general, as is often the case, we have found it less expensive in terms of both capital and labor costs to build complexity into software rather than hardware.

Modularity. Because our development is relatively early-stage, it has been important to organize the system into functional units that can be fabricated, tested, and modified independently prior to integration [2]. The hardware system consists of four primary units: (1) illumination tank, (2) electronics assembly, (3) liquid reservoir station, and (4) computer for image processing. The first three units are integrated into an overall patient interface, but the image-reconstruction computer can be located anywhere; in fact, as part of early-stage development, image reconstruction is often executed off line and off site.

Modularization has also proved useful within the four basic units. This is particularly true of the electronics assembly, where the microwave circuitry is divided into a radio-frequency (RF) switching network, a local-oscillator (LO) power-divider network, and a set of transceiver modules. There are also low-frequency electronics performing digital signal sampling, namely a commercial analog-to-digital (A/D) board plus signal-conditioning unit. In general, we have purchased the highest-quality components affordable. For instance, the Agilent ESG 4432B synthesized RF source provides an accurate, clean, wideband signal and a coherent reference for use at the receiver. The Agilent unit is easily controlled through a general-purpose interface bus, significantly reducing system complexity and integration costs.

Spectral capability. Broadband design requires tradeoffs between cost, response time, size, and other factors. These factors can be particularly difficult to reconcile in cases where the overall bandwidth must be subdivided into narrower bands. Bandwidth also affects antenna design, because antennas generally operate over narrow spectral ranges.

However, broadband capability offers potential benefits for numerical modeling and image reconstruction. Monitoring system performance over a wide bandwidth rather than at a single frequency provides important insight when characterizing installations during early development stages. Furthermore, there may not be an optimal single frequency for breast imaging; rather, different imaging tasks may be best carried out at different frequencies. Reconstructing images at several frequencies simultaneously may also provide benefits. For example, lower-frequency data tends to stabilize image reconstruction and higher-frequency data improves resolution. Multifrequency data may thus improve the ill-conditioning of the inverse problem. Extrapolating the multifrequency concept to its natural limit, we might even reconstruct images in the time domain (with possible increases in diagnostic utility) by Fourier-transforming multifrequency data.

Reliability. We have selected high-speed electrical components having excellent impedance matching, signal-transmission fidelity, and (where appropriate) isolation. This is particularly important in the selection of the amplifiers and switches used in the three microwave-circuit modules. The amplifiers chosen all have a voltage standing-wave ratio (VSWR) of less than 1.25:1 from 300 MHz to 3 GHz and isolation greater than 25 dB. Their high isolation makes them particularly suitable for use as buffers between cascaded components. We have taken care to identify all possible paths of signal leakage and to ensure that all leakage is sufficiently attenuated (e.g., by incorporating extra single-pole, single-throw [SPST] switches) to eliminate channel crosstalk. All component housings are designed with covers having raised surfaces that protrude into the circuit chambers and reduce unwanted signals, and all cables are double-braided to minimize stray radiation.

When appropriate, commercial devices have been purchased to serve certain critical functions. We chose the Agilent synthesized RF source because of its wideband capacity and significant spur rejection in single-sideband modulation mode. Use of this high-end device in a production unit would probably be unnecessary; however, during development it has been imperative to eliminate all potential sources of signal errors so that we can accurately assess our algorithms. Likewise, a National Instruments (NI) A/D board and NI signal-conditioning assembly with programmable gain were purchased as an integrated unit after crosstalk specifications were verified during initial system evaluation. Similar low-risk strategies were used in the design of all modules to assure that they could be fabricated in a timely way.

In the next section, the design and performance of all second-prototype modules are described. The coupling medium, especially with regard to variations in the electrical properties of the breast, is also evaluated. Measured data and images from relevant phantom experiments and patient examinations are reported as well.

2   ELECTRONICS SYSTEM DESIGN AND BREAST INTERFACE

2.1   Superheterodyne Signal Detection

We have chosen a superheterodyne approach to recover the coherent signals required for our reconstruction algorithm [3]. While our operating frequencies (500–3000 MHz) are not particularly high by today's standards, utilizing intermediate frequencies (IFs) of 1 MHz or less has allowed for excellent phase and amplitude detection with relatively low-cost components.

In our calibration scheme, phase and amplitude data are collected both with and without an imaging target present so that the scattered fields for each measurement can be recovered by simple log-magnitude and phase subtractions. Collection of this data generally requires a modulated RF source (i.e., a source offset from a coherent LO reference by the IF frequency) that can be down-converted to produce an IF signal with embedded phase and magnitude information. Two common approaches for producing these RF and LO signal pairs are (1) using two phase-locked signal generators and (2) using one signal generator with a portion of its output coupled to and modulated by a single-sideband up-converter (traditionally an I-Q modulator). The former approach has the attraction that spurious signals do not arise from modulation, but entails the added size and cost of a second generator. In the latter approach, modulation is generally only possible over a modest bandwidth and with nominal rejection of unwanted sideband signals. Fortunately, certain modulated sources designed specifically for testing applications in wireless communications have combined the benefits of both approaches. The Agilent ESG 4432B produces a modulated signal from 250 KHz to 3 GHz with all unwanted spurs suppressed by 60 dB or more below the carrier.

2.2   Multichannel Design

The number of channels used to acquire data can vary widely. At one extreme is the mechanically-rotated, single-transmitter, single-receiver system. In this case, data acquisition can be prohibitively slow, and in our application would be complicated by mechanical translation (and/or rotation) of the transmitter-receiver antenna pair in a liquid bath. The electronics for such a single-port (single input-output) system, however, are the simplest. At the other extreme, one fixes the antennas at all desired transmit and receive positions and controls the radiate/receive patterns electronically. This scheme, besides being more costly, faces a number of unresolved issues: (1) determining the optimal number of antennas, (2) deciding on 2D versus 3D data acquisition, (3) choosing between dual transmit/receive antennas versus dedicated transmit and receive antennas, and (4) optimizing individual antenna design and orientation around the target.

These considerations are clearly interrelated. For example, number of antennas, spacing of antennas about the target, and individual antenna design all affect one another. It has been our experience in both microwave imaging and electrical impedance imaging that image quality degrades rapidly as antenna-to-target distance increases [4]; there is also a need to keep the electrical distance between adjacent illuminators small (for adequate spatial sampling) while minimizing antenna/antenna interactions (which become significant when spacing is too close). Deciding whether antennas should operate as dual-role transmitter/receivers or as dedicated transmitters and receivers further complicates the antenna-array design. Dual-mode operation has the attraction of increasing the amount of measured data—since, for a given degree of antenna spacing, more transmit and receive points are available—but complicates design of the switching electronics by introducing the possibility of unwanted channel-to-channel crosstalk.

Our design is a hybrid of mechanical motion and electronic switching. The antenna array is a horizontal circular ring of 16 vertically-oriented monopole antennas, each a few centimeters in length. The breast to be imaged is positioned pendant inside the ring. Vertical motion of the ring is provided by a Compumotor Series J linear actuator positioned below the tank. This design allows for horizontally two-dimensional data acquisition at multiple vertical positions and can be readily adapted to three-dimensional acquisition by partitioning the array into interleaved subarrays that can be raised and lowered independently. Further, since the monopole antennas have a small horizontal cross-section, two-dimensional spatial sampling density can be readily increased by packing them more closely. Because of their short vertical length (a few centimeters), spatial sampling in the vertical direction can also be fairly fine. Finally, we have chosen to operate the antennas in the dual transmit/receive mode to maximize the amount of data acquired.

Figure 1 shows a schematic of the overall system design. This includes (1) illumination tank with circular array of 16 antennas, (2) NI A/D board with integrated signal-conditioning unit, (3) 16 transceiver modules (only four of which are shown, for simplicity), (4) 1:16 RF switching matrix, (5) 1:16 LO power-divider network, (6) Agilent modulated RF source, and (7) system control computer. Our electronics can accommodate 32 channels, but this capacity has not yet been utilized. The transceiver, RF switching, LO power-divider, and illumination tank modules are discussed in more detail in the following three sections.

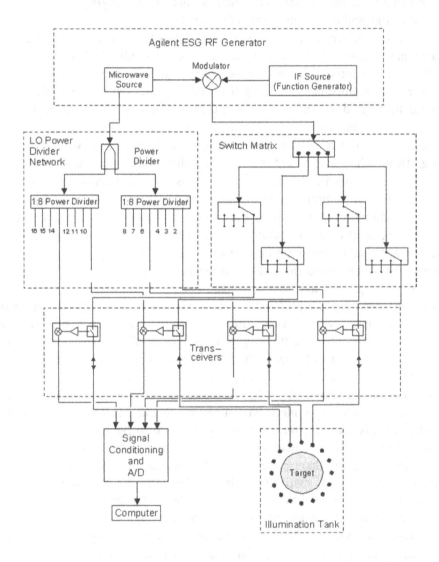

Figure 1. Schematic of the Dartmouth microwave imaging system. For simplicity, only 4 of the 16 signal paths are shown. The switches in the transceiver and switch-matrix modules are always set so that one antenna is selected as a transmitter while the other 15 act as receivers. Control lines from the computer to the various units are not drawn.

2.3   Transceiver Module

Figure 2 shows a schematic of the transceiver module. We chose to implement a separate receiver (i.e., low-noise amplifier [LNA] and mixer) for each channel primarily in order to exploit the parallel-data acquisition capabilities of currently available A/D boards and to minimize channel-to-channel crosstalk. A buffer amplifier (M/A-COM MAAM02350) is positioned at the RF input to boost the power just prior to reaching the antennas. This amplifier (VSWR 1.7:1, isolation 30 dB) damps any mismatch losses from interactions between the components of the switching matrix and the switches in the transceiver. Its isolation characteristics also help to attenuate any spurious signal that might leak backwards through the amplifier into the RF switching matrix and couple to the output of other channels. A second subsection contains an SPST switch (M/A-COM SW05-0311) and a single-pole, double-throw (SPDT) switch (M/A-COM SW10-0312) that select the transmit and receive antenna modes. (The SPDT switch actually performs the mode selection, but the SPST is essential to isolating the transmitting signal from the LNA of the receiver and preventing leakage of the signal back through the RF switching matrix.) Each switch has isolation of 40 to 60 dB over the full operating band.

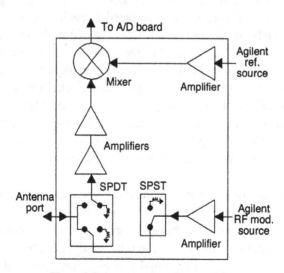

Figure 2. Schematic of receiver module.

On the receiver arm of the module are two LNAs (M/A-COM MAAM02350) and a balanced mixer (Mini-Circuits ADE-30). The LNAs have excellent VSWR to reduce mismatch losses between the switches and mixer, as well as significant isolation to reduce back-leakage to the antenna and switching matrix of various harmonic spurs generated at the mixer. The low noise figure and high gain of each amplifier ($NF = 4.0$, $G = 18$ dB) ensure an excellent cascaded noise figure ($NF_{cascade} = 5.4$) for the composite receiver, which is separated from the antenna by only a single switch. The cascaded noise figure is defined as

$$NF_{cascade} = NF_1 + \frac{NF_2 - 1}{G_1} + \frac{NF_3 - 1}{G_1 G_2} + \cdots \frac{NF_N - 1}{G_1 G_2 \cdots G_{N-1}} \qquad (8.1)$$

where NF_i is the noise figure of the ith cascaded component, G_i is the gain of the ith cascaded component, and N is the number of cascaded stages.

The mixer, which operates over the full band, requires only nominal LO drive power (optimal levels between +7 and +10 dBm) and has a 1 dB compression point of −10 dBm. This enables us to perform linear signal detection from roughly −27 dBm down to the noise floor. At the mixer LO input port is another buffer amplifier (M/A-COM MAAM02350) to suppress signal mismatch losses between the LO power divider network and mixer, boost the LO power prior to mixing, and attenuate any unwanted spurs propagating back through the LO network.

We chose to drive the mixers simultaneously through a power-divider network so that the IF frequencies produced at each channel could be sampled simultaneously for faster overall data acquisition. In such a design, it is important that the drive-power level of the mixer be selected carefully. While the conversion loss of the fundamental received signal will decrease even after achieving a nominal level, the higher-order spurs (most notably, those due to the third and fifth harmonics) increase considerably. In fact, the spurs due to the third and fifth harmonics increase in strength at three and five times the rate of the input power level, respectively, and can quickly reach levels which can contribute significantly to the phase error of the desired signal (Figure 3).

All modules are oriented to minimize loss by keeping transmission paths short. Coplanar waveguides are utilized, where possible, to reduce loss without exciting extraneous cavity (housing) modes. All components are segregated into individual chambers connected by small apertures. These apertures are just large enough to fit the actual transmission lines and act as cutoff waveguides to suppress coupling of cavity-mode signals between chambers. Finally, the housing covers are machined with raised surfaces to minimize coupling of signals into the free space outside the modules.

24-bit A/D boards were not commercially available at reasonable cost when we designed and implemented our second-generation prototype system.

This has changed dramatically, and 24-bit boards are now readily available with sufficient sampling speed and channel count. However, this discussion will focus on the design of our 16-bit system.

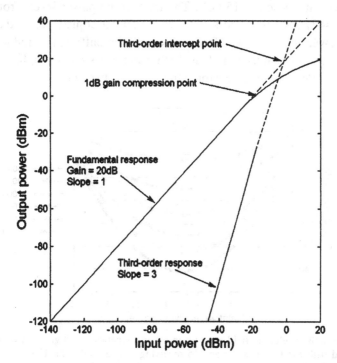

Figure 3. Intercept plot for third-order harmonics. Viable operating range is the linear region of the fundamental response, at left; system design assures that third-order harmonics do not interfere with the operating range (i.e., that the third-order intercept point is sufficiently far to the right).

The receiver design goal was not only to sample signals down to a low noise floor but also to sample the much higher-amplitude signals generally associated with antennas proximal to the transmitter, and to do so over as broad a frequency range as possible. Figure 4 shows simulated signal amplitudes at 15 receiver antennas for a signal broadcast by one transmit antenna in an 80:20 glycerin:water coupling medium over 500 to 2500 MHz. The antennas are mounted on a 15-cm diameter array with relative receiver number 8 being the farthest from the transmitter. Given the free-space loss factor [5], increased attenuation at the higher frequencies, and the broad operating frequency band, it is clear that the effective dynamic range required exceeds the 90 dB range of a 16-bit A/D board. To compensate, we utilized a variable-gain preamplifier (NI SCXI-1125) that allowed us to dynamically increase the gain applied to the IF signal by a factor of 1 to 1000 immediately prior to sampling. We could then sample the weakest signals with the highest gain setting and the strongest signals (generally those from receivers closest to the transmitter) with the lowest. In this way the effective dynamic range of the receiver was increased to 150 dB. The transmitted power levels from the Agilent ESG 4432B synthesized source are computer-adjustable, so that the transmitter power for the lower frequencies can be sufficiently reduced to avoid possible system saturation. This further improves data-sampling capability over the widest possible dynamic range and frequency band.

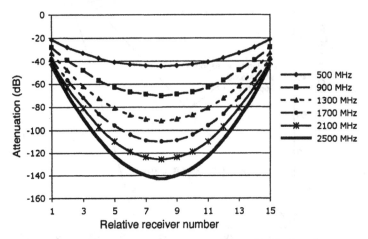

Figure 4. Simulated electric-field strength in a homogeneous 80:20 glycerin:water background bath for 1 transmitter and 15 receiving sites at 500, 900, 1300, 1700, 2100, and 2500 MHz.

Figure 5 shows the power spectrum of a low-amplitude IF signal measured at the A/D converter. The system bandwidth for purposes of computing the theoretical noise floor is 2 KHz, as defined by the IF frequency divided by the full number of IF signal periods sampled by the A/D converter (in this case, 1). The noise floor for this example, as seen at the A/D board, is roughly −120 dBm. (For lower IF frequencies, the noise floor increases due to $1/f$ noise). The effective noise floor for the RF signal at the receiver is considerably lower, due to transmission loss in the SPDT switch, conversion loss in the mixer, and the gains of the two low-noise amplifiers preceding the mixer. For this case, the RF frequency is 1.4 GHz and the cascaded gain is roughly 14 dB. This gain, when combined with the observed −120 dBm IF noise floor, gives an effective RF noise floor of −134 dBm. This is very close to the theoretical limit of −136 dBm when the 5.4 dB noise figure is taken into account. The available thermal noise is −141 dBm at room temperature for a 2 kHz bandwidth.

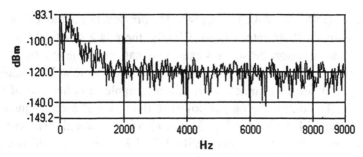

Figure 5. System IF power spectrum in detecting a −110 dBm, 1.4 GHz RF signal (2 KHz IF signal).

2.4   RF Switching and LO Power Divider Networks

Only one antenna at a time illuminates the target; all others act as receivers. This requires a switching network, which we have created by cascading one SPDT switch (M/A-COM SW10-0312) with two levels of single-pole, four-throw (SP4T) switches (M/A-COM SW15-0315) for a combined 1:32 corporate switching matrix. Each switch has a nominal VSWR of 1.5:1 with insertion loss of 1.0 dB or less over the band. The switches' excellent impedance characteristics minimize reflection losses. The channel-to-channel isolation, which is defined in the worst case by the single-switch isolation, is better than 40 dB across the band. Given that these signals are amplified immediately afterward in the transceiver modules, the extra isolation provided by the SPSTs and the SPDTs of the transceiver modules is essential to prevent leakage of the transmitted signal into the receiver circuitry of adjacent channels. The goal of the system is to measure signals down to −130 dB, so inadequately attenuated leakage signals could easily corrupt measurements.

For our second-generation system we wanted to exploit the parallel operation of commercially available A/D boards. This required that the mixers at all receiver channels be driven simultaneously, which we achieved by using a five-level corporate network of two-way power dividers (Sage Laboratories 4122) with two sets of buffer amplifiers (M/A-COM MAAM02350) to boost the output power levels for driving the mixers in the transceiver modules. The Sage power dividers were not optimal for this wideband application, in the sense that their designed operating frequency range was only 1–2 GHz (these types of components are inherently narrowband). Outside this range, the VSWR and isolation of each power divider degraded considerably, while the insertion loss only diminished slightly. In a cascaded configuration without some form of buffering, suboptimal VSWR outside the preferred range can cause significant mismatch losses. We employed well-matched coaxial attenuators (INMET 2A-03) along with the previously mentioned buffer amplifiers to dampen these interactions. Clearly, there is a practical limit to the amount of attenuation between stages that can be achieved by these means; however, 3 dB was generally sufficient, and we were able to realize even output power for all channels with minimal ripple at either end of the frequency band. To control the output power to the mixer at each frequency, a digital attenuator (M/A-COM AT-213) was also incorporated. (The coherent reference source from the Agilent ESG 4432B RF generator did not include an output power-level control.)

2.5   Illumination Tank

Figure 6 shows the illumination tank with antenna array, both in isolation and integrated with the electronics assembly and exam table. Each monopole antenna consists of a vertical, rigid segment of coaxial cable attached to a mounting plate below the tank, which occupies the upper third of the unit. The center conductor of the cable protrudes 3.3 cm above the termination of the outer conductor and is protected by a Teflon sheath. The coaxial rods slide vertically through hydraulic seals in the base of the tank. The mounting plate's vertical position is adjusted by a computer-controlled linear actuator (Compumotor, series J) to allow for data collection at multiple levels. The antennas can operate with minimal artifacts as close as 1 mm from the liquid-air interface, allowing for data collection all the way from the nipple up to near the chest wall. This is important, given the large fraction of cancers detected in the axillary region. One planned improvement is the use of multiple, interleaved arrays to facilitate cross-plane data collection, which will be essential as we proceed to three-dimensional image reconstruction.

The coupling liquid we have chosen is a mixture of glycerin and water. Figure 7 shows the conductivity and relative permittivity of this fluid as functions of frequency. Permittivity levels can be optimized for any frequency range by manipulating the glycerin:water ratio. Given the low permittivity of breast tissue (caused by its high fat content), a relatively low-permittivity coupling fluid is desirable to reduce image artifacts due to large reflections at the breast-fluid interface. As for conductivity, the antennas generally require a coupling medium with $\sigma = 1.0$ S/m or greater for proper operation (to provide them with sufficient resistive loading). Beyond this threshold, however, the extra attenuation associated with greater conductivity

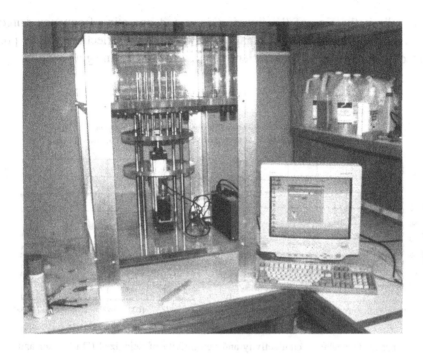

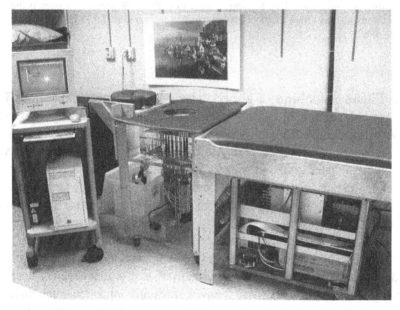

Figure 6. Antennas, illumination tank, and computer-controlled linear actuator assembled on test bench (top) and integrated with breast interface (bottom).

acts to limit the size of the imaging zone and operating frequency range. Since the coupling fluid is attenuating, unwanted tank reflections can be prevented by placing its walls sufficiently far away from the imaging zone.

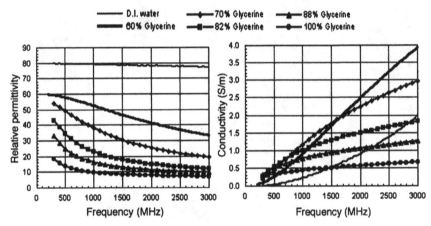

Figure 7. The relative conductivity and permittivity of deionized (D.I.) water and five different mixture ratios of glycerin and water. The 88% glycerin mixture is the one closest to that which we have used in the illumination tank (i.e., a glycerin:water ratio of 87:13).

As Figure 7 confirms, a glycerin:water ratio of approximately 88% is useful for breast imaging because it provides appropriately low permittivity. For this ratio, the conductivity is relatively constant above 1 GHz (i.e., about 1.0 S/m), which compares favorably to the rapidly increasing conductivity of lower glycerin:water ratios. In general, no coupling fluid is ideal for all cases because the electrical properties of individual breasts vary, largely due to their variable fat content. An 87:13 mixture is reasonable for the property range typically encountered.

A glycerin-and-water mixture is used because, in addition to having good electrical properties, it is well-suited to tissue contact. Glycerin is a common ingredient of soaps, hand creams, and many foods; is inexpensive; does not cause any known skin irritations; is environmentally innocuous; and does not support bacterial growth (a significant concern in the clinical setting [4]).

3   RESULTS

Although the published data on *ex vivo* electrical properties of the normal breast are limited and contradictory [6, 7], it is known that over the ultra-high-frequency and microwave ranges the principle parameter determining tissue permittivity and conductivity is water content [8]. Generally, both quantities follow a simple Fricke relationship with respect to tissue water content. Variations are related to amounts of bound water versus free water. The water content of dense fibroglandular tissue can range from 30% to 70%, while that for adipose tissue (most of the breast) is generally under 25% [9]. Furthermore, breast composition varies by individual, with some breasts being mostly adipose while others are largely glandular. Figure 8 shows a series of MR image slices for a healthy breast [10].

To further complicate matters, the physiology of the breast, like that of many other organs, changes significantly with age. The most dramatic changes occur after menopause, when much of the glandular tissue atrophies and is progressively replaced with adipose tissue. Breast physiology also varies notably throughout the menstrual cycle [11].

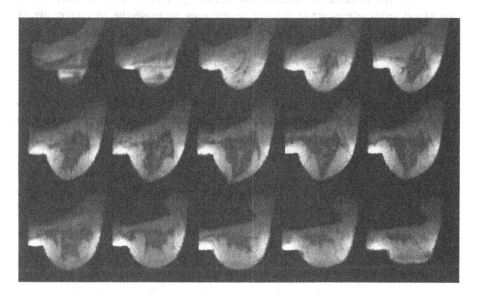

Figure 8. A sequence of anatomically sagittal MR sections of a breast from medial to lateral in 3 cm increments. (Images are ordered left to right in each line, lines are ordered top to bottom.) Dark regions correspond to glandular tissue and light regions to adipose tissue. For these images, the breast was positioned in the vibrating apparatus of the MRE system (i.e., slightly compressed). Internal inhomogeneity is notable.

In vitro tissue is available for refined property measurements. However, Foster and Schepps [8] have shown that *in vivo* breast-tissue properties change with perfusion approximately in accordance with the equation

$$\frac{\varepsilon^* - \varepsilon_r^*}{\varepsilon^* + x\varepsilon_r^*} = p\,\frac{\varepsilon_b^* - \varepsilon_r^*}{\varepsilon_b^* + x\varepsilon_r^*} \tag{8.2}$$

Here, ε_b^*, ε_r^*, and ε^* are the complex permittivities of blood, tissue in the absence of blood, and perfused tissue, respectively; p is the blood-volume fraction; and x is the blood-cell shape factor. For tissues with high water content, such as muscle and most internal organs, the effect of blood volume is minimal, but for adipose and other low-permittivity tissues the effect of blood volume can be significant [8]. Furthermore, blood volume can be an important indicator of tumor activity. In near-infrared spectroscopic imaging, oxygenated hemoglobin is the primary parameter for cancer detection [10]. The physiological basis for this correlation is the increased cellular metabolism and angiogenesis associated with tumor growth. The extra water from the blood volume present at the tumor site may increase the *in vivo* contrast between normal and malignant tissue. A comprehensive study of *in vivo* breast properties would be difficult at this time; therefore, values published for *ex vivo* breast tissue must suffice as a starting point for the clinical imaging problem.

We have primarily investigated the effects of background contrast on reconstructed images of the breast and of phantoms. We have attempted to identify an optimal coupling medium. This is a difficult task, not only because of the factors noted above but because of recently published data suggesting that breast radiographic density has a direct impact on average tissue properties measured *in vivo* [12]. No single medium, therefore, can couple optimally to all breasts. Our studies, along with imaging variations associated with operating frequency and multiple planes of the breast, are reviewed below.

3.1   Raw Data Comparison

Figure 9 shows the 500 MHz scattered-field phases measured at the nine receivers associated with a single transmitter. (Data was acquired from only nine receivers because this study used the first-generation electronics system, which only acquires data at the nine antennas directly opposite to a given transmitter.) These data were acquired in the plane closest to the chest wall of a 53-year-old woman with radiographically scattered breasts. Data were collected for four background media covering a range of contrasts with the breast: (1) 70% glycerin (2) 60% glycerin, (3) 50% glycerin, and (4) 0.9% saline (listed lowest-contrast to highest-contrast). The scattered-field values indicate the degree of difference (in both log-magnitude and phase) between the measured field values when a scattering target is present relative to the homogenous (no-target) situation. In all cases shown in Figure 9, the phase values are largest for receivers 4, 5, and 6 and taper towards 0° at receivers 1 and 9. Since the phase projections are all negative, the average breast dielectric properties are lower than those of the four coupling media used. Additionally, the magnitude of the maximum phase projection is generally well-behaved and increases monotonically with contrast. The values to either side of the projection are not so well-behaved and indicate the presence of more complex diffractive effects, especially at the higher contrasts (i.e., for 50% glycerin and 0.9% saline).

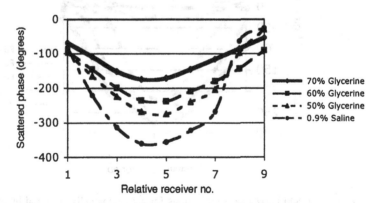

Figure 9. 500 MHz measured phase projections for a radiographically scattered breast in multiple media: (1) 70% glycerin (ε_r = 47.4, σ = 0.61 S/m), (2) 60% glycerin (ε_r = 53.1, σ = 0.87 S/m), (3) 50% glycerin (ε_r = 59.3, σ = 1.25), and (4) 0.9% saline (ε_r = 78.0, σ = 1.59 S/m).

Figure 10 shows the 500 MHz scattered field phase projections for the same patient using the 50% glycerin bath for five coronal planes of the same breast starting nearest the chest wall and separated by 1 cm increments. Interestingly, there is a monotonic reduction in the magnitude of the maximum phase projection with increasing position number. This makes intuitive sense in that the breast's diameter is at a maximum closest to the chest wall and diminishes toward the nipple. The maximum phase projection of each curve in Figure 10 is thus proportional to the planar area transected at each vertical position. In this regard it is interesting to note that the steepest jump in the maximum phase projection occurs between Positions 3 and 4. A photograph of the breast taken during the exam (Figure 11) shows that the transected area shrinks quite abruptly from one plane to the next near the nipple as compared to the more gradual reduction for planes nearer the chest wall.

These qualitative observations generate some confidence that the data reflect the physics of the imaging setup. In addition, they may prove useful in identifying effective plane positions with respect to the geometry of particular breasts. This has generally been difficult to assess by viewing only the reconstructed images, yet is important with regard to cross-correlation analysis of our images and those from the other modalities.

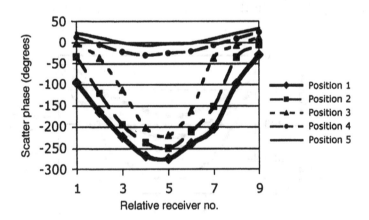

Figure 10. 500 MHz phase projections for a radiologically scattered breast in the 50% glycerin coupling medium for five coronal planes (Positions 1–5) starting closest to the chest wall and separated by 1 cm increments.

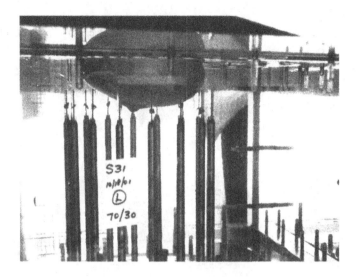

Figure 11. Photograph of a breast pendant in the illumination tank during an exam. Also shown are the partially retracted monopole antennas. The parallax associated with light refraction at the multiple interfaces of plastic and water makes broad feature identification somewhat difficult in this image.

3.2   Contrast Studies

Figure 12 shows recovered 1000 MHz permittivity and conductivity images of a 10 cm diameter homogeneous phantom (i.e., cylinder of molasses, $\varepsilon_r = 15.7$, $\sigma = 0.43$ S/m) immersed in four different background solutions: (1) 0.9% saline ($\varepsilon_r = 76.9$, $\sigma = 1.77$ S/m), (2) 50:50 glycerin:water ($\varepsilon_r = 55.2$, $\sigma = 1.76$ S/m), (3), 60:40 glycerin:water ($\varepsilon_r = 46.7$, $\sigma = 1.48$ S/m), and (4) 70:30 glycerin:water ($\varepsilon_r = 37.4$, $\sigma = 1.28$ S/m). The 16 monopole antennas were positioned on a 15 cm diameter circle with coherent signal detection at 9 opposing antennas for each of the 16 transmitters. First-generation electronics were utilized. Image reconstruction employed the log-magnitude/phase (LMPF) algorithm with a hybrid of the Tikhonov and Marquardt regularization strategies (see Ch. 7). The forward-solution mesh contained 3903 nodes and 7588 triangular elements while the parameter-reconstruction mesh contained 269 nodes and 464 elements.

For the three glycerin:water ratios, the object size, shape, and properties are, as Figure 12 shows, recovered quite well; however, the saline images clearly diverged. The radius, location, and uniformity of the permittivity object component appear to be better than the corresponding conductivity com-

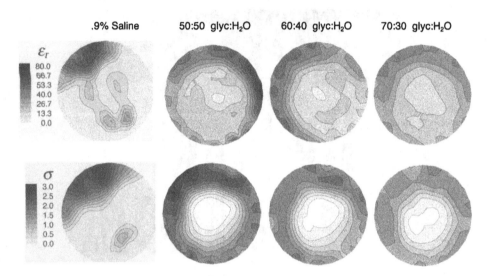

Figure 12. 1000 MHz recovered permittivity (top row) and conductivity (bottom row) images of a 10 cm diameter homogeneous cylinder of molasses, acquired using four backgrounds covering a range of decreasing contrasts: 0.9% saline (first column), 50:50 glycerin:water (second column), 60:40 glycerin:water (third column), and 70:30 glycerin:water (fourth column).

ponents, which are noticeably smaller. As can also be seen, the circular shape of the conductivity object improves progressively with reduced background contrast (more glycerin).

Unwrapped projections of the scattered phase values for a single transmitter for the full range of background contrasts (Figure 13) reveal significant phase wrapping for the saline case. We have demonstrated that this is a possible source of image divergence when utilizing the complex-form algorithm. In extreme cases it can also confound the LMPF approach, since situations can arise where there is not necessarily a unique local phase [13]. That is, the unwrapped phase value at a given point can depend on the path taken in the unwrapping process. This underlines the need to minimize the contrast between breast and background.

Figure 14 shows 1000 MHz permittivity and conductivity images for the same molasses phantom used in Figures 12 and 13, except that the phantom now contains a 3 cm diameter cylindrical saline inclusion in the lower right quadrant. As in the homogeneous molasses phantom experiments, the images diverge for the saline background. For all of the glycerin:water background cases, the phantom structure is well-defined in both the permittivity and conductivity images, with some minor blurring of the recovered permittivity objects into the imaging-zone boundary. The inclusion is readily visible for all of the permittivity images, but its shape is best resolved in the lowest-

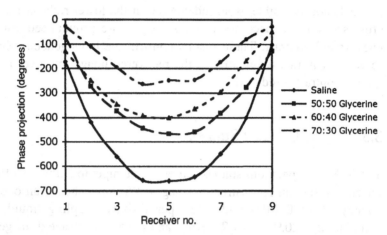

Figure 13. Unwrapped phase projections measured at nine receiver antennas for a single transmitter at 1000 MHz, acquired using four backgrounds covering a range of contrasts. The same phantom was used as in Figure 12.

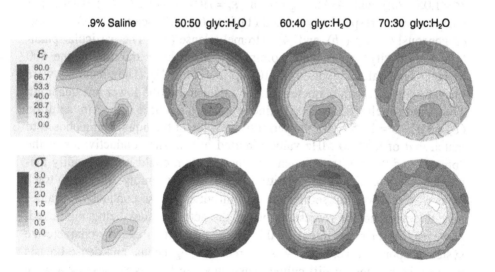

Figure 14. 1000 MHz recovered permittivity (top row) and conductivity (bottom row) images of a 10 cm diameter cylinder of molasses with a 3 cm diameter cylindrical saline inclusion in the lower right quadrant. The images were acquired using four backgrounds covering a range of contrasts: 0.9% saline (first column), 50:50 glycerin:water (second column), 60:40 glycerin:water (third column), and 70:30 glycerin:water (fourth column).

contrast case (70:30). In all three of the glycerin:water conductivity images, the inclusion is visible as an indentation in the lower right of the recovered cross-section that becomes progressively more pronounced with lowered background contrast. These results confirm the homogeneous-phantom observations, in that the quality of the recovered image improves as the background contrast is reduced [14].

3.3   Low-Contrast Studies

The following phantom studies represent attempts to study the effects of reduced contrast on reconstructed images. We have chosen an operating frequency of 1300 MHz and a low-permittivity coupling liquid, i.e., 79% glycerin ($\varepsilon_r = 20.9$, $\sigma = 1.27$ S/m), and have reconstructed images for a 10 cm diameter, thin-walled plastic cylinder containing a variety of breast-mimicking liquids. The phantom mixtures we have devised are glycerin-and-water mixtures containing (1) 97% glycerin ($\varepsilon_r = 8.9$, $\sigma = 0.47$ S/m), (2) 88% glycerin ($\varepsilon_r = 13.1$, $\sigma = 0.83$ S/m), (3) 84% glycerin ($\varepsilon_r = 16.4$, $\sigma = 1.05$ S/m), and (4) 80% glycerin ($\varepsilon_r = 19.9$, $\sigma = 1.18$ S/m). These four phantoms were respectively termed (1) fatty (sf), (2) scattered (ss), (3) heterogeneously dense (sh), and (4) extremely dense (sx). The particular phantom permittivity values were nominally chosen by extrapolating the 600 MHz in vivo values reported in [10] up to 1300 MHz. The phantoms were imaged with a 2.1 cm diameter "tumor" inclusion in the lower left quadrant. The tumor inclusion was a cylinder containing 55% glycerin solution ($\varepsilon_r = 51.1$, $\sigma = 1.45$ S/m), the permittivity value of the liquid being chosen to match that of the 900 MHz value reported in [7]. The conductivities of the "breast" and "tumor" components of the phantom could not be readily manipulated independently of permittivity and so were simply allowed to track what was achieved by setting the permittivities. These conductivity values may therefore not be representative of the actual tissues being mimicked; however, the primary intent of this study was not to exactly characterize system response to actual fatty, scattered, heterogeneous, and dense breasts but to assess potential difficulties when imaging breasts possessing a wide range of property values.

Figure 15 shows 1300 MHz reconstructed images for all four breast phantoms with the tumor-like inclusion in a 80:20 glycerin:water bath ($\varepsilon_r = 20.9$ and $\sigma = 1.27$ S/m). The array of monopole antennas was configured to have a 15 cm diameter, giving an imaging zone of 14.5 cm diameter. The forward-solution finite element mesh had 3903 nodes and 7588 triangular elements, while the reconstruction parameter mesh contained 559 nodes and 1044 elements. The outline of the breast phantom is readily discernable in all cases except that of the *sx* phantom (where failure to resolve the boundary is due to low contrast with the background). As expected, the recovered bulk ε_r and σ values for the phantoms progress monotonically from quite low levels for the *sf* case to being nearly equal to those of the background for the *sx* case. It is notable that the recovered distribution for the conductivity is generally more uneven than the permittivity. We have found this to be a fairly typical observation for many phantom and patient imaging experiments to date. Additionally, the level of artifact is highest in the *sf* case and progressively diminishes toward the *sx* case.

In all cases, the tumor inclusion is well-resolved in both the ε_r and σ images. (The grayscale was deliberately set to allow some recovered values of the tumor inclusion to saturate so that resolution of the remainder of the phantom and background could be readily examined.) The peak values at the center of the recovered inclusions were ε_r = 32.1, 32.1, 31.9, and 39.4 and σ = 1.37, 1.58, 1.58, and 1.57 S/m for the *sf*, *ss*, *sh*, and *sx* cases, respectively. These are good property estimates, considering the inclusion's high contrast with respect to the rest of the phantoms and its relatively small size.

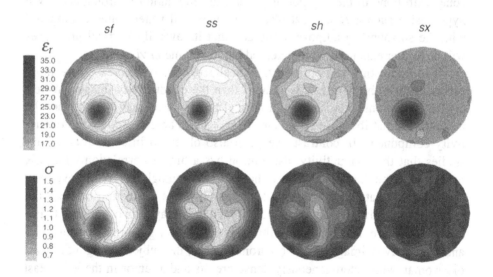

Figure 15. 1300 MHz reconstructed relative permittivity and conductivity images for a 10 cm diameter phantom with a 2.1 cm diameter tumor-like inclusion. The phantom relative permittivity and conductivity values were *sf*: 8.9, 0.47 S/m; *ss*: 13.1, 0.83 S/m; *sh*: 16.4, 1.05 S/m; and *sx*: 19.9, 1.18 S/m.

3.4   Clinical Examples

Figure 16 shows 900 MHz reconstructed permittivity and conductivity images for the right breast of a 45-year-old woman. The images show seven coronal planes positioned at 1 cm increments starting nearest the chest wall. The subject's breasts were radiographically heterogeneously dense. The images are informative in that the recovered cross-sections are largest in diameter nearest the chest wall and diminish as they approach the nipple near plane 7, with the permittivity and conductivity pairs tracking each other well. A dominant feature in the permittivity images is a localized property increase in the lower left quadrant. Although interpreting these images according to standards prevailing in the literature might suggest that this substantial property increase is due to a tumor [7, 13], this woman had normal breasts. We have hypothesized that the increased-permittivity area corresponds to a concentrated zone of fibroglandular tissue.

Figure 17 shows an MR image for a single coronal slice relatively close to the chest wall. There is a large darkened zone oriented towards the lower left. In fact, it occupies approximately half of the total area. While the segregation of tissue types is not absolute (i.e., not all glandular tissue is in one zone, with none in the neighboring area), differentiation is pronounced. We hypothesize such a zone most likely has increased water content compared with the surrounding adipose tissue and that its overall electrical properties will be further enhanced with increased blood volume *in vivo* [15].

It is interesting to note that the localized property increases are more pronounced in the permittivity images than the conductivity images. Water-content variations associated with normal breast tissue may thus impact the permittivity distribution to a greater degree than the corresponding conductivity component. In contrast, we have also observed in some preliminary studies that the conductivity distribution has a higher correlation with NIR recovered hemoglobin [12]. Given that elevated hemoglobin levels have been shown to correlate well with breast tumors [10], this distinction between the recovered permittivity and conductivity images may prove important. For example, Figure 18 shows the 900 MHz left- and right-breast permittivity and conductivity images for two coronal planes, the subject being a 53-year-old woman with heterogeneously dense breasts and a tumor in the left breast as verified by x-ray mammography and confirmed with biopsy. In this case, the fibroglandular regions are readily visible in symmetric lower, outer locations for the contralateral breasts. For the left breast, there is a localized increased permittivity area just above the glandular region at the

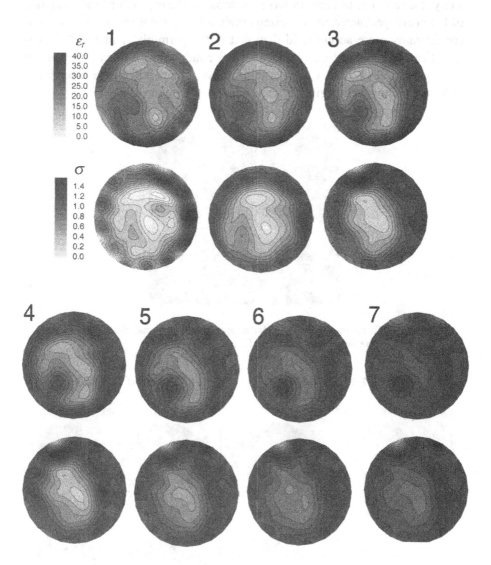

Figure 16. 1100 MHz reconstructed relative permittivity (top of each pair) and conductivity (bottom of each pair) images for the normal, heterogeneously dense right breast of a 45-year-old woman. Images are recorded at seven planes 1 cm apart, ordered from the chest wall to just above the nipple.

known tumor location of about 3 o'clock. While the corresponding conductivity image is not as clear in terms of broad features, such as identification of the breast perimeter, the localized conductivity increase at the tumor site is considerably more accentuated than that in the permittivity image. It is also significantly enhanced compared with the conductivity values observed for the contralateral breast. Understanding these effects will prove essential in utilizing microwave imaging for breast cancer detection.

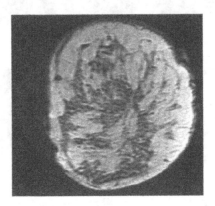

Figure 17. T2 weighted MR image for a representative coronal plane close to the chest wall for the same breast imaged in Figure 16.

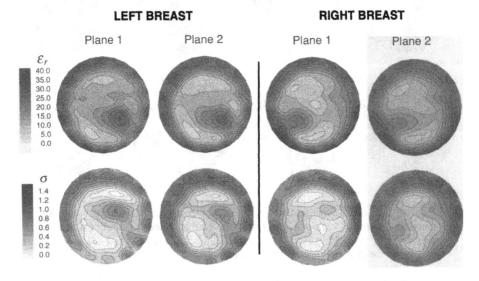

Figure 18. 900 MHz reconstructed permittivity (top row) and conductivity (bottom row) images for the first two planes closest to the chest wall for the left and right breasts of a 53-year-old woman with heterogeneously dense breasts. A tumor is located in the left breast at roughly 3 o'clock, relatively close to the chest wall.

REFERENCES

[1]   D. Li et al., "A parallel-detection microwave spectroscopy system for breast imaging." *IEEE Transactions on Instrumentation*, 2004 (submitted).

[2]   P. M. Meaney et al., "An active microwave imaging system for reconstruction of 2-D electrical property distributions." *IEEE Trans. Biomed. Eng.*, Vol. 42, 1995, pp. 1017–1026.

[3]   M. I. Skolnick, *Introduction to Radar Systems* (New York: McGraw-Hill, 1980).

[4]   A. Hartov et al., "Using multiple-electrode impedance measurements to monitor cryo-surgery." *Med. Phys.*, Vol. 29, 2002, pp. 2806–2814.

[5]   C. A. Balanis, *Antenna Theory: Analysis and Design* (New York: Harper & Row, 1982).

[6]   S. S. Chaudhury et al., "Dielectric properties of normal and malignant human breast tissues at radiowave and microwave frequencies." *Indian J. Biochem. Biophys.*, Vol. 21, 1984, pp. 76–79.

[7]   W. T. Joines et al., "The measured electrical properties of normal and malignant human tissues from 50 to 900 MHz." *Med. Phys.*, Vol. 21, 1994, pp. 547–550.

[8]   K. R. Foster and J. L. Schepps, "Dielectric properties of tumor and normal tissues at radio through microwave frequencies." *J. Micro. Power*, Vol. 16, 1981, 107–119.

[9]   H. Q. Woodward and D. R. White, "The composition of body tissues." *Bri. J. Rad.*, Vol. 59, 1986, pp. 1209–1219.

[10] B. W. Pogue et al., "Quantitative hemoglobin tomography with diffuse near infrared light: Pilot results in the breast." *Radiology*, Vol. 218, 2001, pp. 261–266.

[11] R. Cotran, V. Kumar, and T. Collins, *Robbins Pathologic Basis of Disease, 6th Edition* (Philadelphia: W.B. Saunders Company, 1999).

[12] S. P. Poplack et al., "Electromagnetic breast imaging—average tissue property values in women with negative clinical findings." *Radiology*, Vol. 231, 2004, pp. 571–580.

[13] D. L. Fried and J. L. Vaughn, "Branch cuts in the phase function." *Applied Optics*, Vol. 31, 1992, pp. 2865–2882.

[14] P. M. Meaney et al., "Importance of using a reduced contrast coupling medium in 2D microwave breast imaging." *Journal of Electromagnetic Waves and Applications*, Vol. 17, 2003, pp. 333–355.

[15] H. Q. Woodward and D. R. White, "The composition of body tissues." *Bri. J. Rad.*, Vol. 59, 1986, 1209–1219.

REFERENCES

[1] ...

Chapter 9

NEAR INFRARED SPECTROSCOPIC IMAGING: THEORY

Hamid Dehghani, Ph.D. and Brian Pogue, Ph.D.

1   INTRODUCTION

The propagation of infrared light in tissue is not described by simple, loga-rithmic attenuation, as is the transmission of x-rays, but is approximated as a multiple-scattering transport process [1, 2]. Several groups are seeking to model light propagation in tissue using the diffusion approximation for ra-diation transport and to reconstruct tomographic images from diffuse projec-tion measurements. Diffusion tomography poses two theoretical challenges: (1) derivation of an optical-fluence rate diffusion model that accurately matches the observed light distribution in tissue and the optical flux at its surface (the implementation of such a model is often termed the *forward problem*), and (2) estimation of tissue's optical properties by matching the solution of the forward problem to measurements of the optical flux at the surface (this estimation task is often termed the *inverse problem*). In general, both the forward and inverse problems yield approximate solutions, and small inconsistencies in either can result in degraded image quality.

In this chapter, numerical methods for solving both the forward and in-verse problems are outlined in the context of near-infrared (NIR) spectro-scopic imaging of the human breast. Because our imaging approach is not only multifrequency but tomographic, it is sometimes referred to as near-infrared *tomography*.

In the forward problem, the diffusion equation is generally applicable when

• applied to bulk tissues in which scattering dominates absorption (i.e., most soft mammalian tissues) [3, 4], and

• the point of measurement is more than a few scattering lengths (i.e., in tissue, more than about 3 mm) from the point of illumination [5].

Generally, in any regime where the optical fluence is significantly greater than the directional flux, the diffusion approximation will be adequate.

Within these confines, the choice of the appropriate boundary conditions at the tissue surface has been an issue of particular interest and remains controversial [5–14]. In general, the air-tissue boundary is reasonably approximated by a partial-current or Robin (type III) boundary condition, where the flux at a point on the surface is assumed to be proportional to the fluence rate at that point multiplied by a coupling coefficient. (See (9.2) and (9.3) for definitions of fluence and flux.) The exact value of this coupling coefficient has been the subject of several investigations [5–14]. In our earlier modeling studies, where a two-dimensional finite element (FE) method was applied in NIR tomography [15, 16], we found it useful to derive the coupling coefficient as a free parameter, thus allowing a good empirical fit between the model and the data under homogeneous conditions. However, in the present work, development of a fully three-dimensional FE model facilitates examination of this coefficient beyond its empirical fit to the data, and we investigate how well the theoretically motivated value fits both our model and experimental data [17].

2   FORWARD PROBLEM

2.1   The Diffusion Equation

The derivation of the diffusion equation is briefly recounted below, with an emphasis on how this derivation impacts the FE implementation and the boundary conditions that might be applied.

The interaction of light with tissue is dominated by elastic scattering of photons by cellular organelles, membranes, and structural matrices. The optical radiance in tissue should therefore be well-predicted by the single-velocity radiation transport equation, a form of the Boltzmann equation [18]:

$$\frac{1}{c_m}\frac{\partial L(\mathbf{r},t,\hat{\mathbf{s}})}{\partial t}+\nabla\cdot\hat{\mathbf{s}}\,L(\mathbf{r},t,\hat{\mathbf{s}})$$

$$=-\mu_t L(\mathbf{r},t,\hat{\mathbf{s}})+\mu_s\iint_{4\pi}L(\mathbf{r},t,\hat{\mathbf{s}})f(\hat{\mathbf{s}},\hat{\mathbf{s}}')\,d\Omega'+S(\mathbf{r},t,\hat{\mathbf{s}}) \qquad (9.1)$$

where c_m is the velocity of light in the medium; $L(\mathbf{r},t,\hat{\mathbf{s}})$ is the radiance at point $\mathbf{r}$, time t, and solid angle $\hat{\mathbf{s}}$; $\mu_t = \mu_a + \mu_s$ (where μ_a and μ_s are the absorption and scattering coefficients, respectively, which specify a photon's probability of absorption or scattering per unit distance traveled); $f(\hat{\mathbf{s}},\hat{\mathbf{s}}')$ is the normalized differential scattering function, which predicts the probability of scattering from angle $\hat{\mathbf{s}}'$ into the angle $\hat{\mathbf{s}}$; and $S(\mathbf{r},t,\hat{\mathbf{s}})$ is a source function.

Equation (9.1) is readily simplified to yield the diffusion equation by invoking two assumptions: (1) the radiance is only linearly anisotropic, and (2) the rate of change of the flux is much lower than the collision frequency. The derivation of the diffusion approximation further assumes that the radiance in tissue can be represented by an isotropic fluence rate, $\Phi(\mathbf{r},t)$, plus a small directional flux, $\mathbf{J}(\mathbf{r},t)$, where

$$\Phi(\mathbf{r},t)=\iint_{4\pi}L(\mathbf{r},t,\hat{\mathbf{s}})\,d\Omega \qquad (9.2)$$

and
$$\mathbf{J}(\mathbf{r},t)=\iint_{4\pi}L(\mathbf{r},t,\hat{\mathbf{s}})\hat{\mathbf{s}}\,d\Omega \qquad (9.3)$$

With these two quantities defined, the radiance given by (9.1) can be expanded into a first-order set of spherical harmonics and integrated over all solid angles to give the radiation transport equation:

$$L(\mathbf{r},t,\hat{\mathbf{s}})=\frac{1}{4\pi}\Phi(\mathbf{r},t)+\frac{3}{4\pi}\mathbf{J}(\mathbf{r},t)\cdot\hat{\mathbf{s}} \qquad (9.4)$$

By substituting (9.2) and (9.3) into (9.4) and integrating over all angles, we arrive at the continuity equation for the photon flux:

$$\frac{1}{c_m}\frac{\partial\Phi(\mathbf{r},t,\hat{\mathbf{s}})}{\partial t}+\nabla\cdot\mathbf{J}(\mathbf{r},t,\hat{\mathbf{s}})=-\mu_a\Phi(\mathbf{r},t,\hat{\mathbf{s}})+S_0(\mathbf{r},t) \qquad (9.5)$$

Next, multiplying (9.1) by $\hat{\mathbf{s}}$ and integrating over all angles leads to

$$\frac{1}{c_m}\frac{\partial \mathbf{J}(\mathbf{r},t)}{\partial t} = -\frac{1}{3}\nabla\Phi(\mathbf{r},t) - \frac{1}{3D}\mathbf{J}(\mathbf{r},t) \qquad (9.6)$$

where D is the diffusion coefficient, i.e., $D = 1/[3(\mu_a + \mu_s')]$. (The parameter μ_s' is the *reduced* scattering coefficient, related to the scattering coefficient μ_s by $\mu_s' = (1-g)\mu_s$, where g is the anisotropic factor, equal to 0.9 for biological tissue.) Equation (9.6) can be further simplified, since under most conditions the time derivative of the flux is much less than the collision frequency, i.e.,

$$\frac{1}{\mathbf{J}}\frac{\partial \mathbf{J}}{\partial t} \ll \frac{c_m}{3D} \qquad (9.7)$$

This simplification leads to Fick's Law:

$$\mathbf{J}(\mathbf{r},t) = -D\nabla\Phi(\mathbf{r},t) \qquad (9.8)$$

Equation (9.8) is generally valid for steady-state solutions and time-varying fluxes where the frequency is less than about 1 GHz [19, 20]. The diffusion equation can then be obtained by substituting (9.8) into (9.5):

$$\frac{1}{c_m}\frac{\partial \Phi(\mathbf{r},t)}{\partial t} - \nabla \cdot D\nabla\Phi(\mathbf{r},t) + \mu_a\Phi(\mathbf{r},t) = S_0(\mathbf{r},t) \qquad (9.9)$$

We have been able to achieve an equation that reliably predicts the fluence rate within a highly scattering medium because we have assumed that the radiance is dominated by the isotropic fluence rate and is only weakly anisotropic [1]. It is well-recognized that this equation will not be accurate near boundaries or sources, so it cannot be assumed that diffusion theory will predict measurements near abrupt boundary changes; nonetheless, (9.9) is routinely used to predict the flux exiting from tissue surfaces by applying boundary conditions that allow a relatively good match between calculated and measured data.

We obtain the frequency-domain version of (9.9) by Fourier transforming each term to yield

$$-\nabla \cdot D\nabla\Phi(\mathbf{r},\omega) + \left(\mu_a + \frac{i\omega}{c}\right)\Phi(\mathbf{r},\omega) = S_0(\mathbf{r},\omega) \qquad (9.10)$$

where ω is the intensity modulation frequency of the light signal. The fluence at any point, $\Phi(\mathbf{r},\omega)$, is a complex quantity. Equation (9.10) can be solved for specific regular geometries analytically or for more general shapes using the FE method. Measurements of the optical flux at the boundary can be predicted, using Fick's Law, as the normal derivative of the fluence in the direction of the optical detector:

$$\Phi_m(\mathbf{r},\omega) = -D\hat{\mathbf{n}}\cdot\nabla\Phi(\mathbf{r},\omega) \tag{9.11}$$

Here $\hat{\mathbf{n}}$ is the unit normal vector at the boundary point indexed by m.

2.2   Boundary Conditions

The best description of the air-tissue boundary is given by an index-mismatched Robin-type boundary condition, where the fluence at the surface of the tissue exits and does not return. The flux leaving the boundary is thus equal to the fluence rate at the boundary times a factor that accounts for internal reflection of light back into the tissue [6, 21]. This relationship is described by

$$\Phi(\mathbf{r},\omega) = 2AD\hat{\mathbf{n}}\cdot\nabla\Phi(\mathbf{r},\omega) \tag{9.12}$$

The value of the boundary reflection coefficient, A, depends upon the indices of refraction of tissue and air. (The term A could be redefined to eliminate the factor of 2 in (9.12), but we have not done so in order to be consistent with earlier authors.) Groenhuis et al. [6] derive

$$A \approx \frac{1+r_d}{1-r_d} \tag{9.13}$$

where $r_d = -1.440 n_{rel}^{-2} + 0.710 n_{rel}^{-1} + 0.668 + 0.064 n_{rel}$, n_{rel} being the relative index of refraction of tissue with respect to air. Keijzer et al. [22] use a different approach to define A, deriving it from Fresnel's law as

$$A \approx \frac{\dfrac{2}{1-R_0} - 1 + \left|\cos\theta_c\right|^3}{1 - \left|\cos\theta_c\right|^2} \tag{9.14}$$

where $\theta_c = \arcsin(1/n_{rel})$ is the critical angle and $R_0 = (n_{rel}-1)^2/(n_{rel}+1)^2$.

Both (9.13) and (9.14) yield $A = 1.0$ for a matched boundary (i.e., $n_{rel} = 1.0$), which leads back to (9.12). For a typical tissue-air value of $n_{rel} = 1.33$, we get $A = 2.82$ using (9.13) and $A = 2.34$ using (9.14). For our work, we have adopted the boundary coefficient defined by (9.14).

We model the diffusion equation over a given imaging volume using the FE method, which is attractive due to its geometric flexibility. We generate meshes using the open-source program NETGEN [23]. Figure 1a shows a typical cylindrical mesh of tetrahedral finite elements, with dots added to represent sources and detectors (co-located, in this case). Figure 1b shows the calculated fluence for a single source modeled as a Gaussian point distribution located one scattering distance below the surface at the position indicated by the arrow. As might be expected, the uniform cylindrical target is filled with a diffuse glow that is brightest nearest the source.

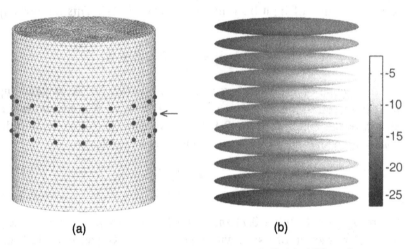

(a)   (b)

Figure 1. Exemplary solution of the forward problem. (a) Cylindrical FE mesh containing 12,587 nodes and 63,857 linear tetrahedral elements. The arrow indicates the location of the source used for this example; other dots represent the remaining 47 sources (unused) and colocated detectors. (b) Calculated log intensity of the fluence throughout the cylinder. Each plane represents a horizontal slice through the mesh.

3   INVERSE PROBLEM

3.1   Problem Statement

In solving the inverse problem in image reconstruction, the goal is to estimate the most accurate possible values of μ_a and μ'_s at each FE node based on a finite number of measurements of optical flux at the tissue surface. Various reconstruction schemes have been employed by members of the imaging community, including (1) analytic methods, (2) back-projection methods, (3) linear methods, and (4) nonlinear methods. For a good overview of these techniques, the reader is referred to Arridge [2].

Most image-reconstruction algorithms seek to minimize an objective function that depends on the difference between the measured data Φ^m and calculated data Φ^c (obtained from a forward solution, as described above). Both Φ^m and Φ^c depend on source and detector position, operating frequency, and the spatial distribution of μ_a and μ'_s. Typically, the objective function to be minimized is

$$\chi^2 = \sum_{i=1}^{O_{IM}} \left(\Phi_i^m - \Phi_i^c \right)^2 \tag{9.16}$$

where i is the index for each source-detector pair and O_{IM} is the total number of measurements. A least-squares minimum of χ^2 can found by setting its derivative equal to zero and using a Gauss-Newton iterative approach to solve the resulting equation (see Ch. 2, Sec. 3.1). In particular, we use a Levenberg-Marquardt algorithm to repeatedly solve the matrix equation

$$\left\{ a \right\} = \left[[J]^T [J] + \lambda [I] \right]^{-1} [J]^T \left\{ b \right\} \tag{9.17}$$

where $\{b\} = \{\Phi^c - \Phi^m\}$ is a vector of length $2O_{IM}$; $\{a\}$ is the solution update vector, length $2L$, which defines the difference between the true and estimated optical properties (both magnitude and phase) at all L property-mesh nodes at each iteration; λ is a scalar factor introduced to stabilize matrix inversion; [I] is the $2L \times 2L$ identity matrix; and [J] is the Jacobian matrix, which we calculate using the adjoint method [24]. The Jacobian, which is $2O_{IM} \times 2L$, has the following form:

$$[J] = \begin{bmatrix} \dfrac{\partial \ln I_1}{\partial D_1} & \dfrac{\partial \ln I_1}{\partial D_2} & \cdots & \dfrac{\partial \ln I_1}{\partial D_L} & \dfrac{\partial \ln I_1}{\partial \mu_{a1}} & \dfrac{\partial \ln I_1}{\partial \mu_{a2}} & \cdots & \dfrac{\partial \ln I_1}{\partial \mu_{aL}} \\[2.5ex] \dfrac{\partial \theta_1}{\partial D_1} & \dfrac{\partial \theta_1}{\partial D_1} & \cdots & \dfrac{\partial \theta_1}{\partial D_L} & \dfrac{\partial \theta_1}{\partial \mu_{a1}} & \dfrac{\partial \theta_1}{\partial \mu_{a2}} & \cdots & \dfrac{\partial \theta_1}{\partial \mu_{aL}} \\[2.5ex] \dfrac{\partial \ln I_2}{\partial D_1} & \dfrac{\partial \ln I_2}{\partial D_2} & \cdots & \dfrac{\partial \ln I_2}{\partial D_L} & \dfrac{\partial \ln I_2}{\partial \mu_{a1}} & \dfrac{\partial \ln I_2}{\partial \mu_{a2}} & \cdots & \dfrac{\partial \ln I_2}{\partial \mu_{aL}} \\[2.5ex] \dfrac{\partial \theta_2}{\partial D_1} & \dfrac{\partial \theta_2}{\partial D_2} & \cdots & \dfrac{\partial \theta_2}{\partial D_L} & \dfrac{\partial \theta_2}{\partial \mu_{a1}} & \dfrac{\partial \theta_2}{\partial \mu_{a2}} & \cdots & \dfrac{\partial \theta_2}{\partial \mu_{aL}} \\[2.5ex] \vdots & \vdots & \ddots & \vdots & \vdots & \vdots & \ddots & \vdots \\[2.5ex] \dfrac{\partial \ln I_{O_{IM}}}{\partial D_1} & \dfrac{\partial \ln I_{O_{IM}}}{\partial D_2} & \cdots & \dfrac{\partial \ln I_{O_{IM}}}{\partial D_L} & \dfrac{\partial \ln I_{O_{IM}}}{\partial \mu_{a1}} & \dfrac{\partial \ln I_{O_{IM}}}{\partial \mu_{a2}} & \cdots & \dfrac{\partial \ln I_{O_{IM}}}{\partial \mu_{aL}} \\[2.5ex] \dfrac{\partial \theta_{O_{IM}}}{\partial D_1} & \dfrac{\partial \theta_{O_{IM}}}{\partial D_2} & \cdots & \dfrac{\partial \theta_{O_{IM}}}{\partial D_L} & \dfrac{\partial \theta_{O_{IM}}}{\partial \mu_{a1}} & \dfrac{\partial \theta_{O_{IM}}}{\partial \mu_{a2}} & \cdots & \dfrac{\partial \theta_{O_{IM}}}{\partial \mu_{aL}} \end{bmatrix} \qquad (9.18)$$

Here, $\partial \ln I_i / \partial D_j$ and $\partial \ln I_i / \partial \mu_{aj}$ define the relationships between the log amplitude of the ith measurement and D and μ_a, respectively, at the jth property-mesh node; $\partial \theta_i / \partial D_j$ and $\partial \theta_i / \partial \mu_{aj}$ define the relationship between the phase of the ith measurement and D and μ_a, respectively, at the jth property-mesh node; O_{IM} is the number of measurements; and L is the number of nodes in the property mesh.

The Jacobian matrix (9.18), also often referred to as the sensitivity or weight matrix, describes the relationship between surface measurements and infinitesimal changes in optical properties throughout the volume modeled by the FE matrix. Figure 2 plots the values of a Jacobian matrix for a model having one source-detector pair. For simplicity, the modeled medium is a flat disc with radius 43 mm, $\mu_a = 0.01$ mm^{-1}, and $\mu_s' = 1.0$ mm^{-1}. The plot shows the relative influence on measurements at the detection point (at right-hand side of circle) of small perturbations in μ_a and D at each location in the image, given a point source (at bottom of circle). As one might expect, perturbations at positions lying more or less between the source and detector have the greatest effect on measurements at the detector.

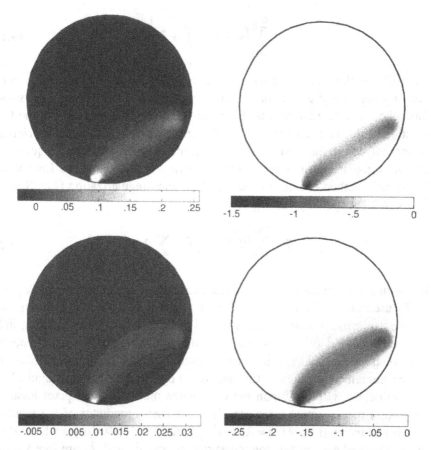

Figure 2. Plots of Jacobian matrix values for a single source-detector pair in a 2D simulation. In all four images, source is at bottom, detector at right. *Top left*: $\partial \ln I_i / \partial D_j$ (i.e., effectiveness of perturbations in D at mesh node j in changing log amplitude measurements at detector i). *Top right*: $\partial \ln I_i / \partial \mu_{aj}$. *Bottom left*: $\partial \theta_i / \partial D_j$. *Bottom right*: $\partial \theta_i / \partial \mu_{aj}$.

3.2   Image Reconstruction

We incorporate regularization methods and *a priori* information into image reconstruction. In theory, both can be included by starting with new objective functions, thereby altering the matrix equation that is solved. In practice, this has been shown to markedly increase the ability to localize and quantitatively characterize objects in tissue-phantom experiments [15].

The Tikhonov approach [25] minimizes an objective variable $\overline{\chi}$, which differs from χ^2 in (9.16) by a penalty term:

$$\overline{\chi} = \sum_{i=1}^{O_{IM}} \left(\Phi_i^m - \Phi_i^c \right)^2 + \lambda \sum_{j=1}^{L} \mu_j^2 \qquad (9.19)$$

Here O_{IM} is the number of measurements, L is the number of nodes in the property mesh, and the regularization parameter λ can, if desired, be varied throughout the iterative process to improve convergence and smooth the final solution [26]. The use of such a penalty term, which may contain *a priori* information about the system, is an attempt to overcome the frequent ill-conditioning of matrices in optical tomography. (Note that the Levenberg-Marquardt method is a special case of Tikhonov regularization [27]. See Ch. 2, Sec. 4.1.) A spatially varying λ, i.e.,

$$\overline{\chi} = \sum_{i=1}^{O_{IM}} \left(\Phi_i^m - \Phi_i^c \right)^2 + \sum_{j=1}^{L} \lambda_j \mu_j^2 \qquad (9.20)$$

has been shown to improve image reconstruction [28]. In this work, Pogue et al. focused on a radially variant regularization (i.e., $\lambda_j = \lambda(r)$), giving λ a simple exponential dependence on radial position in a circular imaging field, i.e., $\lambda(r) = \lambda_0 + \lambda_1 e^{r/10}$. This provided some correction of the radial dependence of imaging field resolution and contrast. More complex distributions can be implemented, such as that suggested by Eppstein and colleagues [29], who calculate λ_j based upon the covariance matrix at each pixel location. Projection measurement error can also be a useful predictor of the regularization parameter (i.e., $\lambda(r) = \lambda_0 + \sigma^2 \lambda_1 [\{\partial\Phi/\partial\mu_s\}^T \{\partial\Phi/\partial\mu_s\}]$, where σ^2 is the variance of each projection measurement and λ_0 and λ_1 are free-varying regularization parameters), thus allowing adaptive regularization based upon the relative uncertainty at each node due to the accuracy of each detector measurement.

If we have structural knowledge of the tissue under investigation (provided by MRI, for example) and estimates of tissue optical properties, we may choose to minimize a modified objective function with some pre-existing distribution μ_0 that incorporates the difference between the current estimate of the optical properties μ subtracted from the initial estimate μ_0. This term can be thought of as a damping factor, which tends to keep the current optical property estimate from straying too far from the initial estimate:

$$\overline{\chi} = \sum_{i=1}^{O_{IM}} \left(\Phi_i^m - \Phi_i^c \right)^2 + \sum_{j=1}^{L} \lambda \left(\mu_j - \mu_0 \right)^2 \qquad (9.21)$$

To calculate this initial optical property distribution input, we use an estimation algorithm similar to that used by Schweiger and Arridge [30], which relies on structural information and boundary data. Tailoring the regularization parameter spatially based upon MRI information leads to the solution

$$\bar{\chi} = \sum_{i=1}^{O_{IM}} \left(\Phi_i^m - \Phi_i^c \right)^2 + \sum_{j=1}^{L} \lambda(r) \left(\mu_j - \mu_0 \right)^2 \qquad (9.22)$$

where $\lambda(r)$ is a function which may be derived from the MR image data. The utility of these functions in characterizing regional heterogeneities appears to be promising.

Finally, in the inverse problem, where we aim to recover internal optical property distributions from boundary measurements, we assume that $\mu_a(r)$ and $\mu_s'(r)$ are expressed in a basis with a limited number of dimensions (less than the dimension of the FE system matrices). A number of different strategies for defining reconstruction bases are possible. In this work we use a second mesh basis whose local shape and continuity characteristics are the same as those used on the original mesh, but with fewer degrees of freedom.

4   IMAGES FROM SIMULATIONS

To illustrate the principles described above, data were simulated for a homogenous cylindrical phantom containing a single absorption anomaly and a single scatter anomaly (Fig. 3). The cylinder has radius 43 mm and height 60 mm and is centered at $(x, y, z) = (0,0,0)$ mm. The mesh contains 12,587 nodes and 63,857 linear tetrahedral elements (see Fig. 1). The background optical properties are $\mu_a = 0.01$ mm^{-1} and $\mu_s' = 1$ mm^{-1}. The absorption anomaly is a sphere of radius 10 mm with $\mu_a = 0.02$ mm^{-1} and $\mu_s' = 1$ mm^{-1}, placed at $(-20,0,5)$ mm. The scatter anomaly is a sphere of radius 10 mm with $\mu_a = 0.01$ mm^{-1} and $\mu_s' = 2$ mm^{-1}, placed at $(20,0,-5)$ mm.

Data were generated using a total of 48 sources and 48 detectors positioned circularly around the FE mesh at $z = -10$, 0, and $+10$ mm. These three levels are denoted by dashed lines in Figure 3. There were 16 sources and 16 detectors per plane. A total of 720 amplitude and 720 phase measurements were calculated (3 planes × 16 sources per plane × 15 detectors per source = 720). In order to simulate realistic measurements, Gaussian noise was added to this data (clipped to maximum 1% of data amplitude range, 2° of data phase range). Absorption and scatter images were calculated using the simulated data and a second mesh was employed for property reconstruc-

tion (see Ch. 2, Sec. 3.2). The absorption and scatter images at the 20th iteration of the reconstruction algorithm are shown in Figure 4. The bright
patches in the absorption and scatter images correspond to the original
anomalies.

Imaging accuracy will be inevitably poorer in planes near the top and
bottom of the cylinder, given their greater distance from the sources and detectors. However, this simulation does demonstrate that our algorithm can (a)
recover a reasonably accurate image from noisy data and (b) distinguish absorption anomalies from scatter anomalies. Images from clinical data and the
extraction of spectral and scattering information from them are discussed in
the next chapter.

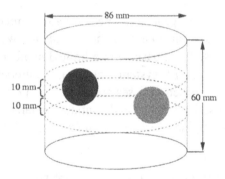

Figure 3. Schematic of model used to generate data for Fig. 4. The absorption coefficient μ_a for the black sphere is twice the background μ_a, and the scattering coefficient μ_s for the gray sphere is twice the background μ_s. Dotted lines indicate
levels at which sources and detectors are positioned at even intervals.

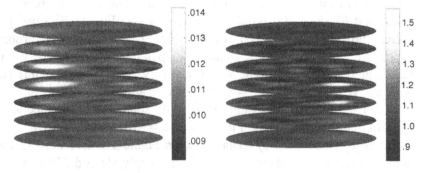

Figure 4. Reconstructed absorption (left) and scatter (right) images for the model in
Fig. 3 (convergence reached at 20th iteration, $\overline{\chi} \leq .01$). Graybar units are mm^{-1}.

5   CALIBRATION

When acquiring patient data, additional data are always measured from a phantom to enable calibration. Precise data calibration is an essential part of image reconstruction [17, 31–33]. The basic steps of calibration are as follows:

1. Using a homogeneous phantom, measurements from all sources in each plane are averaged to produce 15 measurements per plane, $data_{mean}$. Here, both phase and amplitude of the data are used. Since we have a symmetric circular measurement array, $data_{mean}$ is calculated as

$$data_{mean,d} = \frac{1}{N_S} \sum_{n=1}^{N_S} data_{n,d} \qquad (9.23)$$

where d is the number of measurements per source per plane (15 measurements per plane), N_S is the total number of sources per plane, and the data are log amplitude or phase values (see Fig. 6). From this information, global μ_a and μ_s' values are estimated that give the best fit to this data. This is done using a two-step algorithm [32]:

a. Global μ_a and μ_s' values are calculated using an analytical model for an infinite medium coupled to a Newton-Raphson iterative scheme.

b. Using the values calculated in Step 1a as an initial guess, new global μ_a and μ_s' values ($\mu_{a(homog)}$ and $\mu_{s(homog)}'$) are calculated using an FE model of the imaging domain.

2. From the data measured with an anomaly present (i.e., either data from a phantom with a built-in structural anomaly or patient data), Steps 1a and 1b are repeated to calculate global μ_a and μ_s' values for the anomaly data, $\mu_{a(anom)}$ and $\mu_{s(anom)}'$.

3. An offset, $data_{offset(homog)}$ ($3N_S$ points), is calculated between the measured homogenous data, $data_{meas(homog)}$, and the modeled homogenous data, $data_{calc(homog)}$ (the latter calculated using $\mu_{a(homog)}$ and $\mu_{s(homog)}'$). A second offset, $data_{offset(anom)}$, is calculated between the measured anomaly data, $data_{meas(anom)}$, and the modeled anomaly data, $data_{calc(anom)}$ (the latter calculated using $\mu_{a(anom)}$ and $\mu_{s(anom)}'$).

4. Based on the offset values from Step 3 and the homogenous fit, the data are then calibrated using the following relationship:

$$data_{calibrated(anom)} = data_{meas(anom)} - \left(data_{meas(homog)} - data_{calc(homog)}\right)$$
$$- \left(data_{offset(anom)} - data_{offset(homog)}\right) \qquad (9.24)$$

The calibration stage of the reconstruction algorithm eliminates systematic error in the data and provides an initial estimate of the optical properties for image recovery, which is crucial for convergence of the iterative method. The last term in the above equation, $data_{offset(anom)} - data_{offset(homog)}$, corrects for error due to system drift if any exists. In all of our studies, however, this term has been found to be very small.

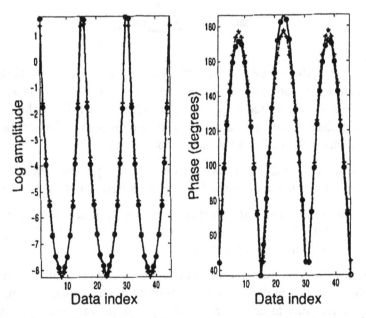

Figure 6. Log amplitude and phase of averaged measured data (dots) compared to averaged calculated data (crosses) for a homogeneous phantom. The calculated data are from an FE forward solution using the global parameter estimates $\mu_{a(homog)}$ and $\mu'_{s(homog)}$. Each 15-point curve (e.g., points 1–15 in the log-magnitude plot) is the averaged data from a single plane. There were 3 planes, thus 45 complex data points. The phantom consisted of Intralipid solution and India ink formed into a cylinder with radius 43 mm and height 100 mm [17].

6   CONCLUSION

In this chapter, the theory behind our modeling and image reconstruction algorithm has been outlined. Implementation of the diffusion equation in a finite element framework has been omitted, as the focus has been on the methods currently in use by our research group. It is important to note that other techniques are widely used for modeling light propagation in media, including analytical, finite difference, and boundary element models. Each has benefits and limitations. For example, although analytical models are computationally faster, they are confined to simple, homogeneous geometries. As for finite-difference models of the diffusion equation, these are conducive to regular grid problems and are not easily implemented for arbitrary shapes (though this can be done). Boundary element models, although not common in this field, again are advantageous when modeling homogenous media.

A common problem in modeling light propagation using the diffusion approximation is implementation of the correct boundary condition. In this chapter discussion has been limited to the type III or Robin ("mixed") boundary condition, as we have found that this option provides the best match between measured and simulated data. Another widely used boundary constraint is the type I condition, which, while not the best practical solution, is easy to implement.

Discussion of image reconstruction has also been limited to the methods and algorithms mostly used by our research group. There are, however, many possible algorithms. A common method is the use of linear or single-step reconstruction, which provides a fast qualitative solution with low quantitative accuracy. Other nonlinear, iterative reconstruction methods exist, such as gradient-based solvers. One benefit of using such algorithms is that the Jacobian does not need to be directly calculated (as in our method) since the cost function itself can be directly derived using the adjoint properties [34]. This allows for more computationally efficient methods. It has been our experience, however, that although gradient-based solvers are computationally faster and require less overhead, they are generally slower to converge to a solution than the algorithm described in this chapter.

It should also be noted that there are a number of methods for calculating the inverse of the Jacobian, which is required for the method described in this chapter. Discussion of these possibilities has been omitted because it has been our experience that the methods described here are adequate. However, the interested reader is referred to the excellent review by Arridge [2].

Finally, simple 3D simulation examples of our modeling and reconstruction algorithm have been included. In the following chapter, the reader can see clinical images that have been obtained using the tools described here.

REFERENCES

[1]   M. S. Patterson et al., "Time resolved reflectance and transmittance for the non-invasive measurement of tissue optical properties." *Appl. Opt.*, Vol. 28, 1989, pp. 2331–2336.

[2]   S. R. Arridge, "Optical tomography in medical imaging." *Inverse Problems*, Vol. 15, 1999, pp. R41–R93.

[3]   B. C. Wilson et al., "The optical absorption and scattering properties of tissues in the visible and near-infrared wavelength range," in *Light in Biology and Medicine*, M. Douglas and Dall'Acqua, eds. Plenum, 1988, pp. 45–52.

[4]   W. F. Cheong et al., "A review of the optical properties of biological tissues." *IEEE J. of Quant. Electr.*, Vol. 26, 1990, pp. 2166–2185.

[5]   T. J. Farrell, M. S. Patterson, and B. C. Wilson, "A diffusion theory model of spatially resolved, steady-state diffuse reflectance for the noninvasive determination of tissue optical properties." *Med. Phys.*, Vol. 19, 1992, pp. 879–888.

[6]   R. A. J. Groenhuis, H. A. Ferwerda, J. J. ten Bosch, "Scattering and absorption of turbid materials determined from reflection measurements. I. Theory." *Appl. Opt.*, Vol. 22, 1983, pp. 2456–2462.

[7]   M. S. Patterson et al., "Diffusion equation representation of photon migration in tissue," in *Microwave Theory and Techniques Symposium Digest*. (IEEE: New York, 1991), pp. 905–908.

[8]   J. X. Zhu, D. J. Pine, and D. A. Weitz, "Internal reflection of diffusive light in random media." *Phys. Rev. A.*, Vol. 44, 1991, pp. 3948–3959.

[9]   I. Freund, "Surface reflections and boundary-conditions for diffusive photon transport." *Phys. Rev. A*, Vol. 45, 1992, pp. 8854–8858.

[10]   C. P. Gonatas et al., "Effects due to geometry and boundary conditions in multiple light scattering." *Phys. Rev. E*, Vol. 48, 1993, pp. 2212–2216.

[11]   R. C. Haskell et al., "Boundary conditions for the diffusion equation in radiative transfer." *J. Opt. Soc. Am. A*, Vol. 11, 1994, pp. 2727–2741.

[12]   A. H. Hielscher et al., "Influence of boundary conditions on the accuracy of diffusion theory in time-resolved reflectance spectroscopy of biological tissues." *Phys. Med. Biol.*, Vol. 40, 1995, pp. 1957–1975.

[13]   R. Aronson, "Boundary conditions for diffusion of light." *J. Opt. Soc. Am. A*, Vol. 12, 1995, pp. 2532–2539.

[14]   J. C. J. Paasschens and G. W. 't Hooft, "Influence of boundaries on the imaging of objects in turbid media." *J. Opt. Soc. Am. A*, Vol. 15, 1998, pp. 1797–1812.

[15]   K. D. Paulsen and H. Jiang, "Enhanced frequency-domain optical image reconstruction in tissues through total-variation minimization." *Appl. Opt.*, Vol. 35, 1996, pp. 3447–3458.

[16]   K. D. Paulsen and H. Jiang, "Spatially varying optical property reconstruction using a finite element diffusion equation approximation." *Med. Phys.*, Vol. 22, 1995, pp. 691–701.

[17]   H. Dehghani et al., "Multiwavelength three-dimensional near-infrared tomography of the breast: Initial simulation, phantom, and clinical results." *Appl. Opt.*, Vol. 42, 2003, pp. 135–145.

[18]   J. J. Duderstadt and L. J. Hamilton, *Nuclear Reactor Analysis* (New York: John Wiley & Sons, 1976), pp. 133–138.

[19]   J. B. Fishkin et al., "Gigahertz photon density waves in a turbid medium: Theory and experiments." *Phys. Rev. E*, Vol. 53, 1996, pp. 2307–2319.

[20]   Moulton, J. D., "Diffusion theory modeling of picosecond laser pulse propagation in turbid media," in *Physics* (McMaster University: Hamilton, 1990).

[21]   M. Schweiger et al., "The finite element model for the propagation of light in scattering media: Boundary and source conditions." *Med. Phys.*, Vol. 22, 1995, pp. 1779–1792.

[22]   M. Keijzer, W. M. Star, and P. R. M. Storchi, "Optical diffusion in layered media." *Appl. Opt.*, Vol. 29, 1988, pp. 1820–1824.

[23]   J. Schöberl, "NETGEN—Automatic mesh generator." Available at http://www.hpfem.jku.at/netgen (accessed Oct. 29, 2003).

[24]   S. R. Arridge and M. Schweiger, "Photon-measurement density functions. Part 2: Finite-element-method calculations." *Appl. Opt.*, Vol. 34, 1995, pp. 8026–8037.

[25]   A. Tikhonov, *Solutions of Ill-Posed Problems* (New York: John Wiley & Sons, 1977).

[26]   A. H. Hielscher and S. Bartel, "Use of penalty terms in gradient-based iterative reconstruction schemes for optical tomography." *J. Biomed. Opt.*, 2001, Vol. 6, pp. 183–192.

[27]   B. Kaltenbacher, "Newton-type methods for ill-posed problems." *Inverse Problems*, Vol. 13, 1997, pp. 729–753.

[28]   B. W. Pogue et al., "Spatially variant regularization improves diffuse optical tomography." *Appl. Opt.*, Vol. 38, 1999, pp. 2950–2961.

[29]   M. J. Eppstein et al., "Biomedical optical tomography using dynamic parameterization and Bayesian conditioning on photon migration measurements." *Appl. Opt.*, Vol. 38, 1999, pp. 2138–2150.

[30]   M. Schweiger and S. R. Arridge, "Optical tomographic reconstruction in a complex head model using a priori region boundary information." *Phys. Med. Biol.*, Vol. 44, 1999, pp. 2703–2722.

[31]   H. Dehghani et al., "Three dimensional optical tomography: Resolution in small object imaging." *Appl. Opt.*, Vol. 42, 2003, pp. 3117–3128.

[32]   T. O. McBride, *Spectroscopic Reconstructed Near Infrared Tomographic Imaging for Breast Cancer Diagnosis*. Ph.D. dissertation, Thayer School of Engineering, Dartmouth College, Hanover, NH, May, 2001.

[33]   T. O. McBride et al., "Strategies for absolute calibration of near infrared tomographic tissue imaging." *Oxygen Transport to Tissue XXIV*, 2003, pp. 85–99.

[34]   S. R. Arridge and M. Schwieger, "Gradient-based optimisation scheme for optical tomography." *Opt. Exp.*, 2(6), 1998, pp. 212–226.

Chapter 10

NEAR INFRARED SPECTROSCOPIC IMAGING: TRANSLATION TO CLINIC

Brian Pogue, Ph.D., Shudong Jiang, Ph.D., Hamid Dehghani, Ph.D., and Keith D. Paulsen, Ph.D.

1   INTRODUCTION

Near-infrared spectroscopic imaging (NIS) has a considerable history in medical applications, ranging from the tremendously successful use of pulse oximetry in critical-care medicine [1] to the failed use of transillumination (diaphanography) of the breast for early detection of cancers [2]. As early as the 1920s, tumors were being examined with red light transmitted through the breast [3, 4]. These investigations were formalized in the 1970s and 1980s with the rapid commercialization of transillumination systems for clinical deployment, even before medical efficacy was established. Studies based on this type of laser scanning for breast imaging continued into the 1980s, culminating in large clinical trials in the US and Sweden [2, 5–8]. Ultimately, transillumination was found not to be as sensitive as mammography, its major limitation being an inability to detect smaller lesions in the breast.

Early attempts to image the breast with near infrared (NIR) light demonstrated certain weaknesses in the approach, yet NIR spectroscopy became very successful. Jobsis discovered that it is possible to measure oxygen-saturation changes in the blood through thick tissue volumes such as the cat cranium [9]. This breakthrough was rapidly exploited for oximetry monitoring of the neonate brain and for measuring arterial oxygen saturation from pulsatile flow in the finger, toe, or earlobe [1, 10–13]. Pulse oximeters have evolved into sophisticated measurement systems that use intelligent methods to suppress movement artifacts, and are now found in most critical-care monitoring settings [1]. The attraction of NIR measurement is the ability to obtain functional information about oxygenation status of the arterial blood with an inexpensive, compact, noninvasive method. NIR monitoring can potentially be extended to methemoglobin, cytochromes [14–19] and their oxygen saturation, and water and lipid content [20]. Similarly, the scattering spectrum and phase function of light in tissue have been shown to provide information about the nuclear transformations from normal tissues to dysplastic or malignant tissues [21–26]. Key to exploiting these potential signatures are (1) continued study of the nature of light scatter and attenuation in tissue, (2) development of advanced technologies for light generation and detection, and (3) appreciation of the heterogeneity existing between subjects and within any given tissue sample.

The interpretation and modeling of light transport in tissue has grown into a sizeable field of study, and understanding of macroscopic light transport in tissue is relatively well-developed. While individual scattering events are well described by direct solution of Maxwell's equations, it has been useful to assume that most scattering centers behave as Mie particles having dimensions similar to the wavelength of the illuminating light. This approach has led to significant new discoveries, e.g., that polarization state and spectral signature preserve information about the scattering-particle size and number density. This offers the diagnostic opportunity to measure cellular characteristics related to volume fraction, nuclear size, and intracellular organelle arrangement.

When light transport is examined more macroscopically, the approximations of radiation transfer become more relevant and the single-energy neutral particle approximation to the Boltzmann equation provides a simple approximation of the transport mechanism [27, 28]. This approach has followed the mathematical formalism of neutron-transport theory, which was largely developed in the 1950s and 1960s [29, 30]. In macroscopic spectroscopy and imaging of tissue with NIR light, this approach allows use of the diffusion equation to model the light transport in tissue. This equation is readily solved both analytically and numerically for a number of different geometries. Numerous studies from the 1980s to the present have focused on the use of analytic solutions from diffusion theory to provide quantitative modeling of light propagation through tissue, demonstrating that this approach can enable deconvolution of absorption and elastic scattering effects. Specifically, the temporal shift of the transmitted light pulse is related to the reduced scattering coefficient of the medium and the exponential decay constant of the tail of the pulse is related to the absorption coefficient of the medium (Figure 1). Patterson et al. [31] demonstrated that the absolute absorption coefficient and the reduced scattering coefficient of a tissue could be analyzed with diffusion-theory solutions. This technique has been extended in many studies to examine frequency-domain light signals [32–35], spatially resolved light signals [36–39], and spectrally resolved light signals [40, 41].

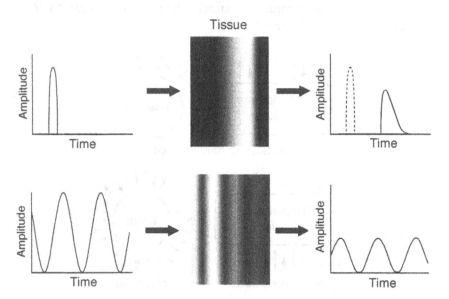

Figure 1. Illustration of a short pulse of light (top) and a sinusoidally modulated beam of light (bottom) being transmitted through a hypothetical block of scattering medium (e.g., tissue). In the pulsed or "time-domain" case (top), the time shift in the peak of the pulse is related to the reduced scattering coefficient, μ_s', and the exponential decay constant of the tail of the pulse is related to the total absorption coefficient of the medium, μ_a [31, 42]. In the amplitude-modulated or "frequency-domain" case (bottom), the signal is attenuated in amplitude and phase-shifted in time. These shifts in the signal can be predicted by diffusion theory, and estimates of μ_s' and μ_a can be derived from them [32, 42, 43].

Numerical solutions to the diffusion equation adequately describe the passage of light signals through irregular tissue regions such as the breast. Thus, diffusion theory based imaging has been developed for numerical image reconstruction [44, 45]. Further theoretical discussion of the diffusion-theory approach is presented in the previous chapter; the remainder of this chapter focuses on the technological and clinical approaches that have been implemented.

2 IMAGING SYSTEM GEOMETRIES: REFLECTANCE, TRANSMISSION, CIRCULAR

Current imaging systems can generally be categorized by their source/sensor geometry. Three specific geometries exist: (1) reflectance for subsurface tomography, (2) parallel-plane projection (transmittance) imaging and tomography, and (3) circular-region or annular tomography. These three geometries are illustrated in Figure 2.

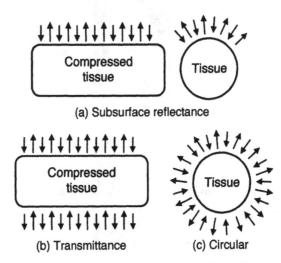

Figure 2. Three NIS imaging geometries: (a) subsurface reflectance, where all source and detection fibers terminate on the upper surface of the tissue (shown at left in a compressed-slab configuration similar to that employed in x-ray mammography); (b) transmittance (with tissue in compressed-slab arrangement); and (c) circular/annular (with sources and detectors distributed evenly around tissue).

The mathematical and computational formalism for NIS image reconstruction was developed by Simon Arridge and David Delpy at University College London [46, 47]. Britton Chance and colleagues at the University of Pennsylvania, together with Enrico Gratton and collaborators at the University of Illinois Urbana-Champaign, pioneered the actual use of reflectance imaging tomography for both brain and breast imaging [48, 49]. Image-reconstruction algorithms were later refined by groups focusing on analytic reconstruction methods [50–54], gradient-based recovery methods, and Newton-type inversion methods [45, 55–63]. The reflectance geometry has been used by several investigators to study brain function, although the limited depth penetration of this approach has led several groups to use this modality for brain "topography" rather than true tomography. This approach has proved successful for studying localized changes in blood volume and oxygen saturation in response to traumas such as stroke or infarct [64–68]. It has also been useful in imaging functional activation changes to determine the normal physiological functioning of the brain [19, 69–72].

In the field of breast imaging, reflectance geometry has been exploited by Chance and colleagues [73] to image palpable breast tumors and by Tromberg and colleagues to record spectra from palpable breast lesions [20, 74, 75]. These studies have made it possible to estimate the available contrast in breast tumors and to gain an initial understanding of the basic spectral signatures of different tumor types. Both Chance et al. and Tromberg et al. chose the frequency-domain approach for its simplicity and reliability.

Breast imaging based on the parallel-plate transmittance geometry typical of radiographic mammography has also been realized. Perhaps the first and most widely discussed system was that developed by Zeiss using algorithms advanced by Fantini and Franceschini [76–78]. Similar systems have been constructed at the University of Pennsylvania, at Massachusetts General Hospital, in Germany, and as a commercial venture by ART Inc. Near-infrared imaging using the parallel-plate geometry continues to be investigated by several researchers for diagnosis of clinically relevant features [79–82]. Fantini et al. continue to analyze the data set from the Zeiss group to determine if oxygen-saturation changes in tumors can be reliably predicted and, if so, whether this provides sufficient information to stage the disease [79, 83].

While the parallel-plate acquisition geometry limits image quality, it provides maximal signal transmission through the breast and thus may provide the best signal-to-noise ratio and, concomitantly, the best information about tumor spectral response. Recent studies by Boas et al. [84] combining NIR imaging with mammography tomosynthesis reconstruction may yield the optimal way to implement this imaging modality in the clinic, especially since the method generates images in the geometry to which mammographers are most accustomed. Further study in this direction would, ideally, be supported by frequency-domain data (for robustness) and iterative image reconstruction methods (for optimal image recovery).

A number of early breast-imaging ventures, including commercial efforts by Phillips Inc. [63, 85] and Imaging Diagnostic Systems (IMDS) Inc. [86, 87], incorporated continuous-wave systems based on a circular geometry [88]. Because these systems were unable to deconvolve absorption and scattering coefficients, they resulted in failed clinical trials. IMDS has made another commercial attempt in this direction using time-resolved data collection and short-pulse laser excitation (http://www.imds.com). Other studies have been conducted by Jiang et al. at Clemson University [89, 90] and by Barbour et al. at the State University of New York [91–95]. In our work at Dartmouth College, the circular geometry has been pursued since 1995, largely because this configuration provides the most symmetric data-collection arrangement and the best sampling of the image space from multiple angles [96]. This, in turn, results in an optimal sampling of the frequency space (K space) for image reconstruction and leads to the optimal spatial frequency distribution. However, it is important to note that the recoverable spatial frequencies are not homogeneous across the image field, so direct comparisons to x-ray tomographic image-reconstruction algorithms are of limited utility. We continue to develop and study NIS imaging in this promising geometry [96].

3   CIRCULAR/ANNULAR TOMOGRAPHY SYSTEM DEVELOPMENT

Initial studies were carried out with tissue-simulating phantoms using a single-source, single-detector system developed at the Hamilton Regional Cancer Center. This led to the successful demonstration of feasibility for NIR imaging in breast-tissue-like media [59, 60, 97–101]. An initial prototype single-channel system was developed at Dartmouth College in 1997 [102] (Figures 3 and 4). This system's success in imaging tissue phantoms led to the development of a first-generation clinical prototype that was tested in a pilot study involving a small group of women [103] including both normal subjects (to characterize variation between subjects) and a few women with characterized tumors. This first-generation system was adapted to feature an array of 32 optical fibers that could be translated radially in and out to accommodate different breast diameters and to facilitate breast positioning within the array. The second-generation array is shown in Figure 4.

We also developed a second-generation light delivery and acquisition system based on serial input of the source and simultaneous parallel detection at all receiver locations [104] (Figure 5). The number of wavelengths was increased to six, which permitted deconvolution not only of oxyhemoglobin and deoxyhemoglobin but also of tissue water fraction [105, 106]. These advances were key to improving the system's ability to accurately quantify the chromophores and scatterers which cause contrast in tumors. In addition, the newest system interface was designed to include three imaging layers, allowing capture of three cross-sections of light data in one setting.

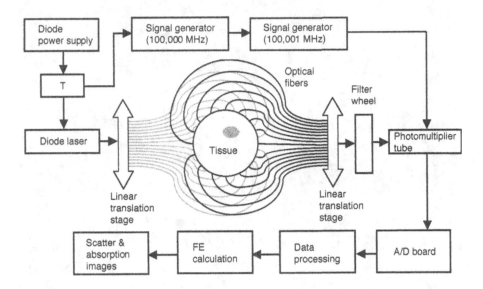

Figure 3. Schematic of NIS tomography system using 16 source fibers (gray) and 16 detection fibers (black). Light from a single laser is launched into the source fibers by sequential alignment of the laser with each fiber using a translation stage. Detection is achieved by aligning a single detector with each fiber using a separate translation stage.

4   CALIBRATION

4.1   System Calibration with Tissue-Simulating Phantoms

For any medical imaging method, the use of tissue-simulating phantoms to evaluate and calibrate the system is central to achieving a useful device. In our studies, we have developed several different types of tissue phantoms, as discussed below.

In all imaging situations, we insert a homogeneous phantom into the fiber array to provide a homogeneous field in which to test the system response and the ability of our finite element code to match the measured data.

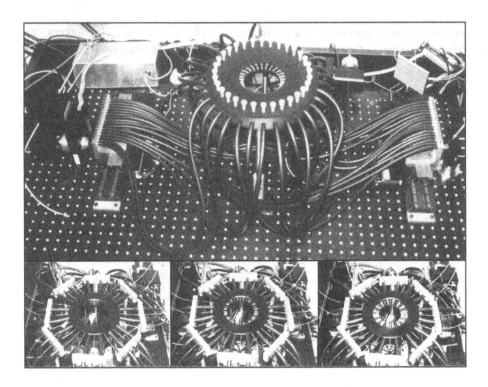

Figure 4. Table-top system (top) whose schematic is shown in Figure 3. In the three photographs at bottom, the first-generation clinical system (schematically similar to the table-top system) is shown with its fibers opened to three different diameters. Each fiber is adjusted one tooth at a time through a mechanical gearing system that simultaneously moves all fibers radially inwards or outwards.

Measurements of phase shift and AC amplitude are taken for the intensity-modulated light that is transmitted through the phantom. These values are averaged for all source positions, assuming that the response at each of the 15 detectors will be the same as the source is rotated (i.e., as each fiber is used in turn as the source). Using this averaged data set, the finite element diffusion simulation is calculated and its absorption and scattering values systematically updated until the best possible approximation is found. In our estimation algorithm, phase shift is treated as a linear function of distance from the source and the slope of this linear relationship is extracted. The same process is completed for the logarithm of the AC amplitude versus distance from the source. These two slopes have been found from both phantoms and tissues to be very robust, and so provide a stable way to fit the

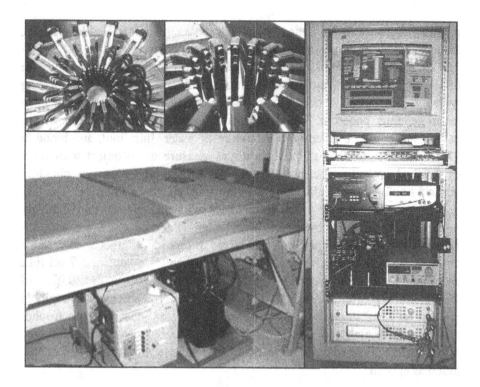

Figure 5. Second-generation system with parallel detection and three layers of optical fibers. The fiber translation array system (top left) drives three layers of fibers (top center) to accommodate radial and vertical positioning relative to the pendant breast. The computer control panel and data acquisition system (right) and the exam table with optical array (bottom left) are also shown. The array of photomultiplier tubes that is translated to multiplex to each of the three layers of 16 detection fibers is immediately below the table.

homogeneous estimates of the bulk optical properties. The fitting of the slopes of phase versus distance and log AC amplitude versus distance is accomplished by a Newton-Raphson algorithm. Estimates of the absorption and reduced scattering coefficients are typically obtained in less than ten iterations. These data are then used in a diffusion-model simulation, along with calculated offsets in AC amplitude and phase shift at zero distance. The best estimate of the simulated data is subtracted from the actual set of measured data and this difference residual is subtracted from all future measurements recorded during the same session. The calibration process provides a correction for interfiber variations in phase and amplitude as well as for any coupling errors. It is important to note that this calibration routine is not equivalent to what is sometimes called "difference imaging" relative to the phantom, because in both cases we match the simulation to the data; hence, the absolute absorption and scattering coefficients are recovered.

We have systematically examined the impact of the properties and size of the homogeneous calibration phantom on image quality by calibrating with different homogeneous phantoms before repeatedly imaging the same heterogeneous phantom. We developed a heterogeneous phantom with a cavity that could be filled with a mixture of water, Intralipid, and blood at varying concentrations, allowing a direct measure of an object with well-established optical properties. Photographs of one heterogeneous phantom and six homogeneous calibration phantoms are shown in Figure 6. The heterogeneous phantom is 84 mm in diameter, with a single, 20 mm–diameter hole parallel to the depth-axis of the cylinder. This hole was filled with different ratios of water, Intralipid, and blood to provide a target with variable contrast. The human blood used in the experiment was kept in a 7 ml tube with liquid additive to reduce the clotting of the platelets (volume, 0.07ml of 15% solution [buffered]; weight: 10.5 mg EDTA[k3]). The total hemoglobin content in these samples of blood was 140 g/dL as measured spectrophotometrically in a clinical co-oximeter system. The blood was then aliquoted into a water-Intralipid solution to make specific concentrations of blood solution as needed.

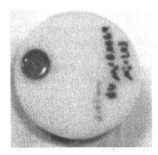 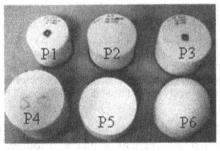

Figure 6. Heterogeneous target phantom (left) and a representative set of homogeneous calibration phantoms (right). The target phantom has a diameter of 84 mm and height of 55 mm, with a cylindrical hole of diameter 20 mm. The homogeneous calibration phantoms labeled P1, P2 and P3 are all 55 mm high but are 73 mm, 84 mm, and 92 mm in diameter, respectively. The average optical property coefficients of P1, P2 and P3 are $\mu_a = .005$ mm^{-1} and $\mu_s' = 1.0$ mm^{-1} for P1; $\mu_a = .005$ mm^{-1} and $\mu_s' = 1.3$ mm^{-1} for P2; and $\mu_a = .004$ mm^{-1} and $\mu_s' = 1.1$ mm^{-1} for P3. Both P4 and P5 were 82 mm in diameter and had $\mu_a = .004$ mm^{-1} and $\mu_s' = 1.6$ mm^{-1}. The P6 phantom is approximately breast-shaped and constructed of a soft, RTV-based material. The bottom diameter and the height of P6 are 82 mm and 78 mm, respectively, and its optical properties are $\mu_a = .0046$ mm^{-1} and $\mu_s' = 1.2$ mm^{-1}.

The phantom's optical properties were measured before the hole was drilled. It was found to have an absorption coefficient (μ_a) of 0.0064 mm^{-1} and a reduced scattering coefficient (μ_s') of 1.0 mm^{-1}, respectively, at a wavelength of 785 nm. The hole was filled with an Intralipid and ink solution which matched the background reduced scattering coefficient and had a slightly higher absorption (0.00643 mm^{-1}) before different concentrations of blood were added. This type of phantom is constructed using the methods described by Firbank et al. [107]. Specifically, 330 grams of resin (GY502 Araldite resin, D. H. Litter, Elmsford, NY) are mixed with 99 grams of hardener (HY832, D. H. Litter), 1.4 g of titanium dioxide, and 0.5 ml of a 2% ink solution. The ingredients are carefully mixed, then degassed in a large bell jar before being moved to an evacuation fume hood to cure for several days. When this process is complete, the phantom is finished by machining (on a lathe) to reduce its diameter to the desired size. Machining is also a good way to reduce the superficial sticky layer that remains after curing. The final product has a solid, smooth surface and is easily handled in the lab.

Measurements from six homogenous phantoms were used to calibrate data recorded from the target heterogeneous phantom. The first three calibration phantoms (P1, P2, and P3 in Figure 6) were constructed from the resin composition discussed above and were similar in composition to the heterogeneous phantom used in this study.

A second kind of phantom was also investigated—a "soft" phantom that provides an elastic property similar to most breast tissue. Coupling of the optical fibers to harder phantoms is never achieved with complete and even contact because the surface is curved and rigid, whereas the ends of the fibers are large and flat. It was, therefore, hypothesized that a softer phantom would provide better contact and thus mimic imaging of the actual breast. A soft, RTV-based material was used to make three soft calibration phantoms (P4, P5, and P6 in Figure 6). These phantoms were fabricated by using 500g Silicone (RTV141, Medford Silicone, Medford, NJ) mixed with 17 g of hardener (comes with RTV141), 1.7 g of titanium dioxide, and 0.8 ml of a 2% ink solution.

Following measurements on all of these phantoms, images of the single inhomogeneous phantom were reconstructed. The absorption coefficient was varied for the inhomogeneous phantom by varying the blood concentration. Values for the slope of absorption coefficient versus blood concentration of an embedded inclusion at a wavelength of 785 nm were compared between data sets reconstructed with calibration phantoms of different stiffness, size, shape, and optical properties. Figure 7 shows plots of the estimated maximum μ_a within the blood region the of target phantom versus blood concentration, with each line of data corresponding to a different homogeneous calibration phantom. The blood concentration was varied from 0% to 1%, as shown on the horizontal axis.

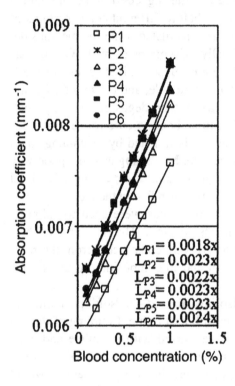

Figure 7. Estimated μ_a versus blood concentration. The lines L_{P1} through L_{P6} are linear regression fits to the values of maximum μ_a within the blood region for phantoms P1 through P6 (see Fig.6). The equations in the lower right-hand corner show the slopes of the fitted lines.

The standard deviation of the slopes of the lines in Figure 7 was 8% of the average slope. If reconstructions from data calibrated using the hard phantom with a diameter of 73 mm (P1) were omitted, the standard deviation was less than 3%. For the variations in the reconstructed absorption coefficient for the same blood concentration, the variations in the reconstructed absorption coefficient for the same blood concentration were within 2% when ignoring the P1 phantom. This shows that the effect of using different calibration phantoms is small as long as all of the source and detector fibers remain in good contact with the target (not the case with P1). Considering the tradeoff between detector size and the curvature of the reference phantom surface, 80–90 mm diameter phantoms with optical properties similar to those of the normal breast appear to produce the best image quality for the 6 mm diameter fiber bundles currently in use within our imaging system. In addition, it can be seen that the μ_a corresponding to the breast-shaped calibration phantom (P6) is approximately the same as the data corresponding to the soft phantom P4, which has the same diameter and similar optical properties and height.

4.2   Calibration of Spectral Absorption Parameters

The measurements recorded by our system at six different wavelengths can, in theory, be used to estimate various chromophore concentrations. (A chromophore is a blood fraction or constituent that possesses distinct optical properties, e.g., red blood cells, lipid bodies, or plasma.) We have, therefore, carried out a series of phantom experiments which test our ability to quantify chromophore concentration changes.

To validate the values of Hb_T (total hemoglobin), S_tO_2 (tissue hemoglobin oxygen saturation), and water concentration obtained by our system and to understand the relationship between the number of wavelengths used and the estimation accuracy, experiments involving a series of phantoms with well-characterized properties were conducted. Reconstructed absorption coefficient images were obtained from the measurements and Hb_T, S_tO_2, and water concentration were estimated for each phantom. The basic phantom was a circular plastic container 90 mm in diameter and 200 mm high. It was filled with Intralipid and human blood in solution at varying blood concentrations, where the Intralipid was fixed at 1.4% to maintain $\mu_s' = 1.5$ mm^{-1} at 785 nm. The blood concentration was varied in successive tests from 0.2% to 1.2% to provide a target with variable contrast. We used the same blood that was employed during the homogeneous phantom calibration testing. Figure 8 shows a set of representative images of the total hemoglobin (Hb_T), oxygen saturation (S_tO_2), water concentration, scattering amplitude, and scattering power within a phantom having a blood concentration of 0.8%.

Images can be formed by implementing a linear inversion to solve for concentrations of total oxyhemoglobin, deoxyhemoglobin, and water based upon knowledge of the molar absorption coefficients and the estimated (imaged) μ_a at all six wavelengths. (This method is described in detail in the following section.) In the images shown here, the edges are effected by the wall of the container and generate lower concentration values than those in the center of the image. Figure 9 shows Hb_T, S_tO_2, and water concentration versus blood concentration from 0.2% to 1.2% when the fitted curves are based on images reconstructed for three, four, five, and six wavelengths, respectively. The solid lines show the true values of Hb_T, S_tO_2, and water

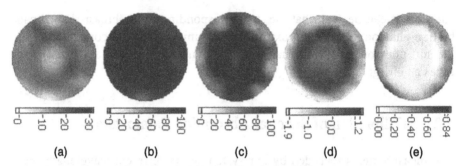

Figure 8. Images of total hemoglobin in units of microMolar (a), tissue oxygen saturation as a percentage (b), water concentration as a percentage of the tissue volume (c), scattering logarithm of amplitude (d), and scattering power (e) are shown for a phantom with a blood concentration of 0.8% in a background solution of 1.4% Intralipid. These images show a ring around the perimeter, which is nominally attributed to the tissue phantom container and which is excluded when we quantify the chromophore or scatterer values in these homogeneous test cases.

concentration within the phantom based upon knowledge of its composition. Three-wavelength fitting utilized 785 nm, 805 nm, and 826 nm. When four, five, and six wavelengths were used for fitting, μ_a values at wavelengths of 761 nm, 661 nm, and 850 nm were added serially to the fitting process. The effect of the walls of the phantom container presents a problem in analyzing this data; to avoid wall effects, all of the values in the analysis were obtained by averaging over a centered circular area with a diameter of 70 mm.

The five- or six-wavelength fits for μ_a are closer to the true values for all three properties (Hb_T, S_tO_2, and water concentration) than those fitted at three or four wavelengths (see Figure 9). The differences between the five- or six-wavelength values for Hb_T, S_tO_2, and water concentrations are 3 μM, 1%, and 1%, respectively. Further studies are ongoing to determine the value of using even more wavelengths in the fitting process.

5   SPECTRAL ANALYSIS OF ABSORPTION IN TISSUE

A unique feature of NIS imaging is its ability to provide information about different absorbing molecules and scatterers within the tissue. When spectral analysis is performed on NIS data (assuming that a sufficient number of wavelengths are measured), several chromophores can be deconvolved.

In single-point measurement systems such as the one demonstrated by Tromberg et al. [108], it is relatively easy to sample multiple wavelengths

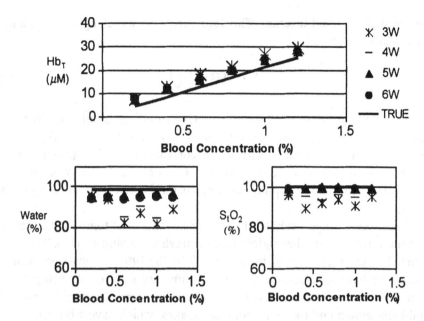

Figure 9. Estimated values of Hb_T (top), S_tO_2 (bottom left), and water concentration (bottom right) as calculated from three, four, five, and six wavelengths of image data are shown for blood concentrations varying from 0.2% to 1.2%. The solid lines show the true values of Hb_T, S_tO_2, and water concentration in the phantom.

in order to solve for the concentrations of various chromophores. The absolute absorption coefficient μ_a at any wavelength λ_k can be calculated from a diffusion-theory analysis; this coefficient can be represented as a linear summation of the absorptions due to all relevant chromophores in the sample, the ith chromophore having molar absorption coefficient $\varepsilon_i(\lambda_k)$ at the kth wavelength:

$$\mu_a(\lambda_k) = \sum_{i=1}^{N_c} \varepsilon_i(\lambda_k) c_i, \quad k = 1, \ldots N_w \qquad (10.1)$$

where there are N_w wavelengths and N_c chromophores and c_i is the concentration of the ith chromophore.

When this spectral analysis is applied to tomographically reconstructed images, it requires that a number of estimates of $\mu_{a,j}(\lambda_k)$ be obtained for each pixel in the image (index j indicates pixel number). Thus, given a set of $\varepsilon_i(\lambda_k)$ values for the N_c relevant chromophores and all relevant frequencies, the inverse of (10.1) must be calculated to determine the array of c_i estimates at every pixel location. This leads, for each wavelength λ_k, to a matrix equation

$$\{c\} = [E]^{-1}\{\mu_a\} \qquad (10.2)$$

where $\{c\}$ is the vector of chromophore concentrations at all pixel locations (length $N_c \times N_p$, where N_p is the number of pixels); $[E]$ is the $N_c N_p \times N_p$ matrix containing the molar extinction coefficients $\varepsilon_i(\lambda_k)$ (having many zero entries) for each of the N_c chromophores at the kth wavelength; and $\{\mu_a\}$ is the vector of absorption coefficients (at the given wavelength) for all pixels.

Based on this approach, we have used multispectral tomographic data to estimate images of oxyhemoglobin and deoxyhemoglobin *in vivo*. The noise in the absorption-coefficient images prohibits the fitting of water concentration, so we have analyzed much of the preliminary *in vivo* data using an average assumed water concentration. These results were then used to calculate total-hemoglobin and oxygen-saturation images, which have a broader applicability for interpreting physiologic and pathophysiologic changes in the breast.

Representative images are shown in Figure 10 for a patient with a 3 cm ductal carcinoma (central right region of each image). The tumor can be clearly seen as a region of increased absorption and increased hemoglobin and water in the spectrally constructed images. Figure 11 presents the images from the contralateral breast of the same patient; no remarkable features are evident in this normal breast tissue. In the latter case, interestingly, there are significant features in the absorption images, but when the spectral analysis is completed these are found to be wavelength-independent and therefore not strongly apparent in the hemoglobin, oxygen-saturation, or water-concentration images. This observation supports the idea of analyzing the clinical significance of the chromophore images rather than absolute absorption-coefficient images. In the chromophore images, the spectral changes must agree with the known spectral absorption of the chromophore or else they do not appear, providing some spectral filtering and thereby reducing artifacts that may only appear at a few wavelengths.

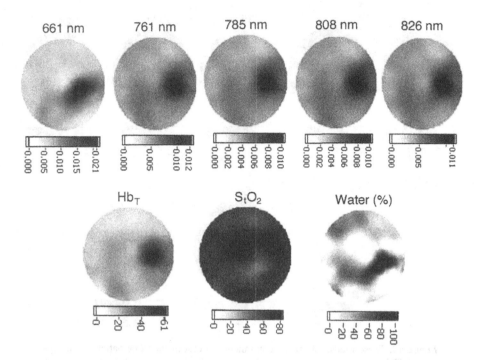

Figure 10. The top row shows multispectral absorption coefficient images for a patient with a ductal carcinoma in the middle right region of the breast cross-section presented here (units of mm^{-1}). The images at bottom report total hemoglobin (Hb$_T$), tissue hemoglobin oxygen saturation (S$_t$O$_2$), and water concentration, respectively.

6   SPECTRAL ANALYSIS OF SCATTERING IN TISSUE

The scattering spectrum provides data about the nature of the scattering particles and, hence, some information on the composition of the tissue. Since scattering in tissue occurs predominantly from Mie-sized particles, the general trend for scattering coefficients is a smooth decrease with increasing wavelength. This curve is well-represented by a power law of the type [22, 107]

$$\mu_a(\lambda) = SA \; \lambda^{-SP} \tag{10.3}$$

where *SA* and *SP* are arbitrary fitting constants for scattering amplitude and scattering power, respectively. *SP* increases with decreasing scatterer size,

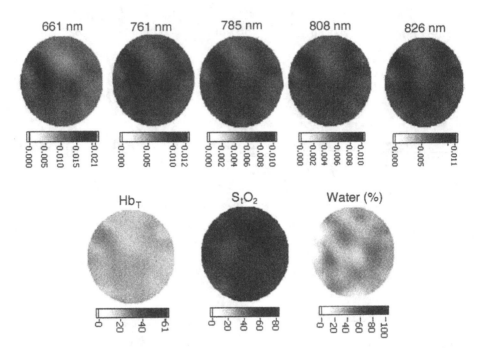

Figure 11. These images show the contralateral breast of the same patient as in Figure 10. This breast is disease-free. It shows considerably lower values in the images of Hb_T, S_tO_2, and water concentration (bottom row).

i.e., as scattering tends toward a Rayleigh spectrum ($SP = 4.0$). As the scattering particle dimension becomes much greater than λ, then the value of SP decreases toward zero. In tissue, typical SP values range between 0.1 and 0.3 [109, 110]. In standard 1% Intralipid solutions used to mimic the scattering of soft tissues, $SP = 0.24$.

In our studies, we have begun to fit the scattering spectrum at each pixel within the image to (10.3) and create images of scattering power and logarithm of the scattering amplitude. A set of representative images is shown in Figure 12 for the patient with an interior ductal carcinoma (same patient as for Figs. 10 and 11). The area of increased scattering can be observed at all wavelengths (top row), as can the effect on scattering amplitude and power (bottom row). In particular, there is a focal increase in amplitude and a focal decrease in scattering power. Images from the contralateral breast are highlighted in Figure 13 for comparison. There are no significant findings in this normal breast.

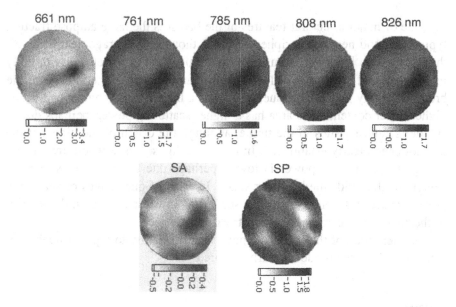

Figure 12. In the top row of images, the reduced scattering coefficient is shown for the same breast presented in Figure 10, which has a localized invasive ductal carcinoma. The two lower images show the logarithm of the scattering amplitude (*SA*) and the absolute scattering power (*SP*), respectively.

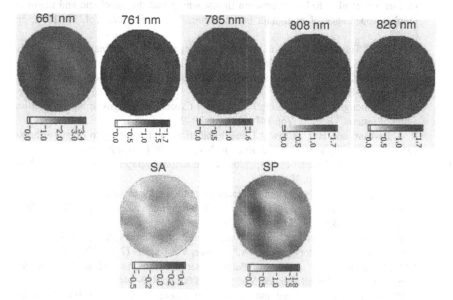

Figure 13. In the top row of images, the reduced scattering coefficient is shown for the contralateral breast of the same patient as in Figures 10–12. The two images at bottom show the logarithm of the scattering amplitude (*SA*) and absolute scattering power (*SP*) for this breast.

One of major structural features of the breast is the large adipose fraction typically found near the periphery. This is thought to average near 75%, although there is large variation between women that is correlated with body mass index and breast size [111–113]. In many instances, the interior of the breast is largely glandular tissue, which has a higher blood content and hence higher water content. This area has a higher scattering power, perhaps due to smaller scattering sites in the tissue, although the origin of the higher value has not been clearly established. In areas of adipose tissue where fat content is high the scattering power is lower, perhaps due to the larger scattering centers of the lipid-filled cellular space. In most of our images of scattering power we see this trend clearly: the scattering power is highest in the interior of the breast and decreases towards its exterior surface.

Further study of the scattering power and its ability to report valuable information about the tissue is clearly required.

REFERENCES

[1]   J. G. Webster, ed., *The Design of Pulse Oximeters*, Medical Science Series (Philadelphia: Institute of Physics Publishers, 1997).

[2]   O. Jarlman et al., "Relation between lightscanning and the histologic and mammographic appearance of malignant breast tumors." *Acta Radiol.*, Vol. 33, 1992, pp. 63–68.

[3]   M. Cutler, "Transillumination as an aid in the diagnosis of breast lesions." *Surg. Gyn. Obst.*, Vol. 48, 1929, pp. 721–729.

[4]   C. H. Cartwright, "Infra-red transmission of the flesh." *J. Opt. Soc. Am.*, Vol. 20, 1930, pp. 81–84.

[5]   D. J. Watmough, "Transillumination of breast tissues: factors governing optimal imaging of lesions." *Radiol.*, Vol. 147, 1982, pp. 89–92.

[6]   R. J. Bartrum and H. C. Crow, "Transillumination light scanning to diagnose breast cancer: a feasibility study." *Am. J. Roentg.*, Vol. 142, 1984, pp. 409–414.

[7]   G. A. Navarro and A. E. Profio, "Contrast in diaphanography of the breast." *Med. Phys.*, Vol. 15, 1988, pp. 181–187.

[8]   A. Alveryd et al., "Lightscanning versus mammography for the detection of breast cancer in screening and clinical practice. A Swedish multicenter study." *Cancer: Diag. Treat. Res.*, Vol. 65(8), 1990, pp. 1671–1677.

[9]   F. F. Jobsis, "Non-invasive, infra-red monitoring of cerebral and myocardial oxygen sufficiency and circulatory parameters." *Science*, Vol. 198, 1977, pp. 1264–1267.

[10]   P. M. Middleton and J. A. Henry, "Pulse oximetry: evolution and directions." *International Journal of Clinical Practice*, Vol. 54(7), 2000, pp. 438–444.

[11]   J. W. Severinghaus, "History and recent developments in pulse oximetry." *Scandinavian Journal of Clinical & Laboratory Investigation—Supplement*, Vol. 214, 1993, pp. 105–111.

[12]   Y. Mendelson, "Pulse oximetry: Theory and applications for noninvasive monitoring." *Clinical Chemistry*, Vol. 38(9), 1992, pp. 1601–1607.

[13] W. A. Bowes et al., "Pulse oximetry: a review of the theory, accuracy, and clinical applications." *Obstetrics & Gynecology*, Vol. 74(3, Pt. 2), 1989, pp. 541–546.

[14] M. Tamura et al., "The simultaneous measurements of tissue oxygen concentration and energy state by near-infrared and nuclear magnetic resonance spectroscopy." *Advances in Experimental Medicine & Biology*, Vol. 222, 1988, pp. 359-63.1988.

[15] S. Wray et al., "Characterization of the near infrared absorption spectra of cytochrome aa3 and haemoglobin for the non-invasive monitoring of cerebral oxygenation." *Biochem. Biophys. Acta*, Vol. 933, 1988, pp. 184–192.

[16] H. Miyake et al., "The detection of cytochrome oxidase heme iron and copper absorption in the blood-perfused and blood-free brain in normoxia and hypoxia." *Analytical Biochemistry*, Vol. 192(1), 1991, pp. 149–155.

[17] H. R. Heekeren et al., "Noninvasive assessment of changes in cytochrome-c oxidase oxidation in human subjects during visual stimulation." *Journal of Cerebral Blood Flow & Metabolism*, Vol. 19(6), 1999, pp. 592–603.

[18] W. Bank and B. Chance, "Diagnosis of defects in oxidative muscle metabolism by non-invasive tissue oximetry." *Molecular & Cellular Biochemistry*, Vol. 174(1–2), 1997, pp. 7–10.

[19] A. Villringer and B. Chance, "Non-invasive optical spectroscopy and imaging of human brain function." *Trends in Neurosciences*, Vol. 20(10), 1997, pp. 435–442.

[20] A. E. Cerussi et al., "Sources of absorption and scattering contrast for near-infrared optical mammography." *Academic Radiology*, Vol. 8(3), 2001, pp. 211–218.

[21] A. H. Hielscher, J. R. Mourant, and I. J. Bigio, "Influence of particle size and concentration on the diffuse backscattering of polarized light from tissue phantoms and biological cell suspensions." *Appl. Opt.*, Vol. 36(1), 1997, pp. 125–135.

[22] J. R. Mourant et al., "Mechanisms of light scattering from biological cells relevant to noninvasive optical tissue diagnostics." *Appl. Opt.*, Vol. 37(16), 1998, pp. 3586–3593.

[23] J. R. Mourant, T. M. Johnson, and J. P. Freyer, "Characterizing mammalian cells and cell phantoms by polarized backscattering fiberoptic measurements." *Appl. Opt.*, Vol. 40(28), 2001, pp. 5114–5123.

[24] V. Backman et al., "Detection of preinvasive cancer cells." *Nature*, Vol. 406(6791), 2000, pp. 35–36.

[25] R. S. Gurjar et al., "Imaging human epithelial properties with polarized light-scattering spectroscopy." *Nature Medicine*, Vol. 7(11), 2001, pp. 1245–1248.

[26] A. Wax et al., "Determination of particle size by using the angular distribution of backscattered light as measured with low-coherence interferometry." *Journal of the Optical Society of America, A: Optics, Image Science, & Vision*, Vol. 19(4), 2002, pp. 737–744.

[27] W. M. Star, J. P. A Marijnissen, and M. J. C. van Gemert, "Light dosimetry in optical phantoms and in tissues: I. Multiple flux and transport theory." *Phys. Med. Biol.*, Vol. 33(4), 1988, pp. 437–454.

[28] M. S. Patterson, B. C. Wilson, and D. R. Wyman, "The propagation of optical radiation in tissue: I. Models of radiation transport and their application." *Lasers Med. Sci.*, Vol. 6, 1990, pp. 155–168.

[29] E. M. Gelbard, "Spherical harmonic methods," in *Computing Methods in Reactor Physics* (New York: Gordon and Breach, 1964).

[30] J. J. Duderstadt and L. J. Hamilton, *Nuclear Reactor Analysis* (New York: John Wiley and Sons, 1976), pp. 133–138.

[31]   M. S. Patterson and B. C. Wilson, "Time resolved reflectance and transmittance for the non-invasive measurement of tissue optical properties." *Appl. Opt.*, Vol. 28, 1989, pp. 2331–2336.

[32]   M. S. Patterson et al., "Frequency-domain reflectance for the determination of the scattering and absorption properties of tissue." *Appl. Opt.*, Vol. 30(24), 1991, pp. 4474–4476.

[33]   J. Fishkin et al., "Diffusion of intensity modulated near infrared light in turbid media." *Proc. SPIE*, Vol. 1431, 1991, pp. 122–135.

[34]   J. B. Fishkin and E. Gratton, "Propagation of photon-density waves in strongly scattering media containing an absorbing semi-infinite plane bounded by a straight edge." *J. Opt. Soc. Am. A*, Vol. 10(1), 1993, pp. 127–140.

[35]   J. B. Fishkin et al., "Gigahertz photon density waves in a turbid medium: Theory and experiments." *Phys. Rev. E*, Vol. 53(3), 1996, pp. 2307–2319.

[36]   T. J. Farrell, M. S. Patterson, and B. C. Wilson, "A diffusion theory model of spatially resolved, steady-state diffuse reflectance for the noninvasive determination of tissue optical properties." *Med. Phys.*, Vol. 19(4), 1992, pp. 879–888.

[37]   A. Kienle and M. S. Patterson, "Determination of the optical properties of semi-infinite turbid media from frequency-domain reflectance close to the source." *Phys. Med. Biol.*, Vol. 42(9), 1997, pp. 1801–1819.

[38]   A. Kienle and M. S. Patterson, "Improved solutions of the steady-state and the time-resolved diffusion equations for reflectance from a semi-infinite turbid medium." *J. Opt. Soc. Am. A—Optics & Image Science*, Vol. 14(1), 1997, pp. 246–254.

[39]   A. Kienle and M. S. Patterson, "Determination of the optical properties of turbid media from a single Monte Carlo simulation." *Phys. Med. Biol.*, Vol. 41(10), 1996, pp. 2221–2227.

[40]   S. J. Matcher and C. E. Cooper, "Absolute quantification of deoxyhaemoglobin concentration in tissue near infrared spectroscopy." *Phys. Med. Biol.*, Vol. 39, 1994, pp. 1295–1312.

[41]   C. E. Cooper et al., "The noninvasive measurement of absolute cerebral deoxyhaemoglobin concentration and mean optical pathlength in the neonatal brain by second derivative near infrared spectroscopy." *Pediat. Res.*, Vol. 39, 1996, pp. 32–38.

[42]   S. R. Arridge, M. Cope, and D. T. Delpy, "The theoretical basis for the determination of optical pathlengths in tissue: Temporal and frequency analysis." *Phys. Med. Biol.*, Vol. 37(7), 1992, pp. 1531–1560.

[43]   B. W. Pogue and M. S. Patterson, "Frequency domain optical absorption spectroscopy of finite tissue volumes using diffusion theory." *Phys. Med. Biol.*, Vol. 39, 1994, pp. 1157–1180.

[44]   J. R. Singer et al., "Image reconstruction of the interior of bodies that diffuse radiation." *Science*, Vol. 248, 1990, pp. 990–993.

[45]   S. R. Arridge and M. Schweiger, "Image reconstruction in optical tomography." *Phil. Trans. R. Soc. Lond. B*, Vol. 352, 1997, pp. 717–726.

[46]   S. R. Arridge et al., "Reconstruction methods for infrared absorption imaging." *Proc. SPIE*, Vol. 1431, 1991, pp. 204–215.

[47]   S. R. Arridge, M. Schweiger, and D. T. Delpy, "Iterative reconstruction of near infrared absorption images." *Proc. SPIE*, Vol. 1767, 1992, pp. 372–383.

[48]   E. Gratton et al., "A novel approach to laser tomography." *Bioimaging*, Vol. 1, 1993, pp. 40–46.

[49]   S. Nioka et al., "Optical imaging of human breast cancer." *Advances in Experimental Medicine and Biology*, Vol. 361, 1994, pp. 171–179.

[50] M. A. O'Leary et al., "Experimental images of heterogeneous turbid media by fre-
      quency-domain diffusing-photon tomography." *Opt. Lett.*, Vol. 20(5), 1995, pp.
      426–428.

[51] D. A. Boas et al., "Detection and characterization of optical inhomogeneities with dif-
      fuse photon density waves: A signal-to-noise analysis." *Appl. Opt.*, Vol. 36, 1997, pp.
      75–92.

[52] D. Boas, "A fundamental limitation of linearized algorithms for diffuse optical tomo-
      graphy." *Opt. Express*, Vol. 1(13), 1997, pp. 404–413.

[53] W. Cai et al., "Time-resolved optical diffusion tomographic image reconstruction in
      highly scattering turbid media." *Proceedings of the National Academy of Sciences of
      the United States of America*, Vol. 93(24), 1996, pp. 13561–13564.

[54] S. Walker, S. Fantini, and E. Gratton, "Image reconstruction by backprojection from
      frequency-domain optical measurements in highly scattering media." *Appl. Opt.*, Vol.
      36(1), 1997, pp. 170–179.

[55] S. R. Arridge and M. Schweiger, "Inverse methods for optical tomography," in *Infor-
      mation Processing in Medical Imaging*, H. H. Barrett, ed. (Flagstaff, AZ: Springer-
      Verlag, 1993), pp. 259–277.

[56] S. R. Arridge and M. Schweiger, "Sensitivity to prior knowledge in optical tomo-
      graphic reconstruction." *Proc. SPIE*, Vol. 2389, 1995, pp. 378–388.

[57] S. R. Arridge, "Optical tomography in medical imaging." *Inverse Problems*, Vol.
      15(2), 1999, pp. R41–R93.

[58] H. Jiang and K. D. Paulsen, "A finite element based higher-order diffusion approxima-
      tion of light propagation in tissues." *Proc. SPIE: Optical Tomography, Photon Migra-
      tion, and Spectroscopy of Tissue and Model Media*, 1995.

[59] H. B. Jiang et al., "Simultaneous reconstruction of optical-absorption and scattering
      maps in turbid media from near-infrared frequency-domain data." *Optics Letters*, Vol.
      20(20), 1995, pp. 2128–2130.

[60] B. W. Pogue et al., "Initial assessment of a simple system for frequency domain diffuse
      optical tomography." *Phys. Med. Biol.*, Vol. 40, 1995, pp. 1709–1729.

[61] K. D. Paulsen and H. Jiang, "Spatially varying optical property reconstruction using a
      finite element diffusion equation approximation." *Med. Phys.*, Vol. 22(6), 1995, pp.
      691–701.

[62] A. H. Hielscher, A. Klose, and K. M. Hanson, "Gradient-based iterative image recon-
      struction scheme for time-resolved optical tomography." *IEEE Trans. Med. Imaging*,
      Vol. 18(3), 1999, pp. 262–271.

[63] S. B. Colak et al., "Tomographic image reconstruction from optical projections in
      light-diffusing media." *Appl. Opt.*, Vol. 36(1), 1997, pp. 180–213.

[64] C. D. Kurth, J. M. Steven, and S. C. Nicolson, "Cerebral oxygenation during pediatric
      cardiac surgery using deep hypothermic circulatory arrest." *Anesthesiology*, Vol.
      82(1), 1995, pp. 74–82.

[65] S. R. Hintz et al., "Bedside imaging of intracranial hemorrhage in the neonate using
      light: comparison with ultrasound, computed tomography, and magnetic resonance im-
      aging." *Pediatric Research*, Vol. 45(1), 1999, pp. 54–59.

[66] E. M. Nemoto, H. Yonas, and A. Kassam, "Clinical experience with cerebral oximetry
      in stroke and cardiac arrest." *Critical Care Medicine*, Vol. 28(4), 2000, pp. 1052–1054.

[67] W. G. Chen et al., "Hemodynamic assessment of ischemic stroke with near-infrared
      spectroscopy." *Hangtian Yixue Yu Yixue Gongcheng/Space Medicine & Medical En-
      gineering*, Vol. 13(2), 2000, pp. 84–89.

[68]   Q. Zhang et al., "Study of near infrared technology for intracranial hematoma detection." *Journal of Biomedical Optics*, Vol. 5(2), 2000, pp. 206–213.

[69]   A. Kleinschmidt et al., "Simultaneous recording of cerebral blood oxygenation changes during human brain activation by magnetic resonance imaging and near-infrared spectroscopy." *J. Cereb. Blood Flow Met.*, Vol. 16, 1996, pp. 817–826.

[70]   H. Obrig et al., "Near-infrared spectroscopy: does it function in functional activation studies of the adult brain?" *International Journal of Psychophysiology*, Vol. 35(2–3), 2000, pp. 125–142.

[71]   B. M. Mackert et al., "Non-invasive single-trial monitoring of human movement-related brain activation based on DC-magnetoencephalography." *NeuroReport*, Vol. 12(8), 2001, pp. 1689–1692.

[72]   C. E. Elwell et al., "Oscillations in cerebral haemodynamics. Implications for functional activation studies." *Advances in Experimental Medicine & Biology*, Vol. 471, 1999, pp. 57–65.

[73]   B. Chance, "Near-infrared (NIS) optical spectroscopy characterizes breast tissue hormonal and age status." *Academic Radiology*, Vol. 8(3), 2001, pp. 209–210.

[74]   B. J. Tromberg et al., "Non-invasive measurements of breast tissue optical properties using frequency-domain photon migration." *Phil. Trans. R. Soc. Lond. B*, Vol. 352, 1997, pp. 661–668.

[75]   N. Shah et al., "Noninvasive functional optical spectroscopy of human breast tissue." *Proceedings of the National Academy of Sciences of the United States of America*, Vol. 98(8), 2001, pp. 4420–4425.

[76]   S. Fantini et al., "Frequency-domain optical mammography: Edge effect corrections." *Med. Phys.*, Vol. 23, 1996, pp. 149–157.

[77]   H. Jess et al., "Intensity modulated breast imaging: Technology and clinical pilot study results." In *Proceedings of the Advances in Optical Imaging and Photon Migration*, *Opt. Soc. Am.*, 1996.

[78]   M. A. Franceschini et al., "Frequency-domain techniques enhance optical mammography: initial clinical results." *Proc. Nat. Acad. Sci USA*, Vol. 94(12), 1997, pp. 6468–6473.

[79]   E. L. Heffer and S. Fantini, "Quantitative oximetry of breast tumors: a near-infrared method that identifies two optimal wavelengths for each tumor." *Appl. Opt.*, Vol. 41(19), 2002, pp. 3827–3839.

[80]   K. Suzuki et al., "Quantitative measurement of optical parameters in normal breasts using time-resolved spectroscopy: In vivo results of 30 Japanese women." *J. Biomed. Opt.*, Vol. 1(3), 1996, pp. 330–334.

[81]   R. Cubeddu et al., "Effects of the menstrual cycle on the red and near-infrared optical properties of the human breast." *Photochemistry & Photobiology*, Vol. 72(3), 2000, pp. 383–391.

[82]   V. Quaresima, S. J. Matcher, and M. Ferrari, "Identification and quantification of intrinsic optical contrast for near-infrared mammography." *Photochem. Photobiol.*, Vol. 67, 1998, pp. 4–14.

[83]   S. Fantini et al., "Performance of N-Images and spectral features in frequency-domain optical mammography." In *SPIE Technical Abstract Digest* (SPIE Press, 1999).

[84]   T. J. Brukilacchio et al., "Instrumentation for imaging of breast lesions based on co-registered diffuse optical and x-ray tomography." *OSA Biomed. Top. Meetings, Technical Digest*, Vol. SuE2, 2002, pp. 178–180.

[85]   J. Hoogenraad et al., "First results of the Phillips optical mammoscope." *Proc. SPIE*, Vol. 3194, 1997.

[86] R. J. Grable et al., "Optical computed tomography for imaging the breast: First look." *Proc. SPIE*, Vol. 4082, 2000.

[87] R. J. Grable, N. A. Gkanatsios, and S. L. Ponder, "Optical mammography." *Appl. Radiol.*, Vol. 29, 2000, pp. 18–20.

[88] P. C. Jackson et al., "The development of a system for transillumination computed tomography." *Brit. J. Radiol.*, Vol. 60, 1987, pp. 375–380.

[89] H. B. Jiang, "Optical image reconstruction based on the third-order diffusion equations." *Optics Express*, Vol. 4(8), 1999, pp. 241–246.

[90] Y. Xu et al., "Three-dimensional diffuse optical tomography of bones and joints." *J. Biomed. Opt.*, Vol. 7(1), 2002, pp. 88–92.

[91] R. L. Barbour et al., "A perturbation approach for optical diffusion tomography using continuous-wave and time resolved data." In *Medical Optical Tomography: Functional Imaging and Monitoring*, G. Muller, ed. (Bellingham,WA: SPIE Publishers, 1993), pp. 87–120.

[92] H. L. Graber, R. Aronson, and R. L. Barbour, "Nonlinear effects of localized absorption perturbations on the light distribution in a turbid medium." *J. Opt. Soc. Am. A, Optics Image Science and Vision*, Vol. 15(4), 1998, pp. 834–848.

[93] C. H. Schmitz et al., "Instrumentation for fast functional optical tomography." *Rev. Sci. Instr.*, Vol. 73(2), 2002, pp. 429–439.

[94] W. Zhu et al., "Iterative total least-squares image reconstruction algorithm for optical tomography by the conjugate gradient method." *J. Opt. Soc. Am. A*, Vol. 14(4), 1997, pp. 799–807.

[95] W. W. Zhu et al., "A wavelet-based multiresolution regularized least squares reconstruction approach for optical tomography." *IEEE Trans. Med. Imag.*, Vol. 16(2), 1997, pp. 210–217.

[96] B. W. Pogue et al., "Comparison of imaging geometries for diffuse optical tomography of tissue." *Opt. Exp.*, Vol. 4(8), 1999, pp. 270–286, 1999.

[97] H. Jiang et al., "Optical image reconstruction using frequency-domain data: simulations and experiments." *J. Opt. Soc. Am. A*, Vol. 13(2), 1996, pp. 253–266.

[98] H. B. Jiang et al., "Frequency-domain optical image reconstruction in turbid media: An experimental study of single-target detectability." *Applied Optics*, Vol. 36(1), 1997, pp. 52–63.

[99] H. B. Jiang, "Frequency-domain fluorescent diffusion tomography: a finite-element-based algorithm and simulations." *Applied Optics*, Vol. 37(22), 1998, pp. 5337–5343.

[100] H. B. Jiang, et al., "Improved continuous *light diffusion imaging in single- and multi-target tissue-like phantoms.*" *Phys. Med. Biol.*, Vol. 43(3), 1998, pp. 675–693.

[101] H. B. Jiang et al., "Frequency-domain near-infrared photo diffusion imaging: Initial evaluation in multitarget tissuelike phantoms." *Med. Phys.*, Vol. 25(2), 1998, pp. 183–193.

[102] B. W. Pogue et al., "Instrumentation and design of a frequency-domain diffuse optical tomography imager for breast cancer detection." *Opt. Express*, Vol. 1(13) 1997, pp. 391–403.

[103] B. W. Pogue et al., "Quantitative hemoglobin tomography with diffuse near-infrared spectroscopy: Pilot results in the breast." *Radiology*, Vol. 218(1), 2001, pp. 261–266.

[104] T. O. McBride et al., "Development and calibration of a parallel modulated near-infrared tomography system for hemoglobin imaging in vivo." *Rev. Sci. Instr.*, Vol. 72(3), 2001, pp. 1817–1824.

[105]   T. O. McBride et al., "Multi-spectral near-infrared tomography: A case study in compensating for water and lipid content in hemoglobin imaging of the breast." *J. Biomed. Opt.*, Vol. 7(1), 2001, pp. 72–79.

[106]   T. O. McBride et al., "Near-infrared tomographic imaging of heterogeneous media: A preliminary study in excised breast tissue." *Proc. SPIE*, Vol. 4250, 2001.

[107]   M. Firbank, M. Oda, and D. T. Delpy, "An improved design for a stable and reproducible phantom material for use in near-infrared spectroscopy and imaging." *Phys. Med. Biol.*, Vol. 40, 1995, pp. 955–961.

[108]   B. J. Tromberg et al., "Non-invasive in vivo characterization of breast tumors using photon migration spectroscopy." *Neoplasia*, Vol. 2(1–2), 2000, 26–40.

[109]   S. Srinivasan et al., "Interpreting hemoglobin and water concentration, oxygen saturation, and scattering measured by near-infrared tomography of normal breast in vivo." *Proceedings of the National Academy of Sciences of the United States of America*, Vol. 100(21), 2003, pp. 12349–12354.

[110]   B. W. Pogue et al., "Characterization of hemoglobin, qater and NIR scattering in breast tissue: Analysis of inter-subject variability and menstrual cycle changes." *J. Biomed. Opt.*, Vol. 9(3), 2004, pp. 541–552.

[111]   H. Vorherr, "Fibrocystic breast disease: pathophysiology, pathomorphology, clinical picture, and management." *American Journal of Obstetrics & Gynecology*, Vol. 154(1), 1986, pp. 161–179.

[112]   S. J. Graham et al., "Quantitative correlation of breast tissue parameters using magnetic resonance and X-ray mammography." *British Journal of Cancer*, Vol. 73(2), 1996, pp. 162–168.

[113]   C. S. Poon et al., "Quantitative magnetic resonance imaging parameters and their relationship to mammographic pattern." *Journal of the National Cancer Institute*, Vol. 84(10), 1992, pp. 777–781.

Chapter 11

STATISTICAL METHODS FOR ALTERNATIVE IMAGING MODALITIES IN BREAST CANCER CLINICAL RESEARCH

Tor D. Tosteson, Sc.D.

1   INTRODUCTION

The imaging modalities that are the focus of this book are being developed to improve the diagnosis and treatment of breast cancer. Essential to this process is research to facilitate the practical application of the new techniques and to identify ways to maximize their clinical utility. In particular, statistical methods can help to establish quantitative measures of imaging and diagnostic accuracy based on data generated by clinical research. In this chapter, several important statistical issues associated with clinical applications and research are explored and illustrated with examples drawn from active projects within the Dartmouth alternative imaging program.

In all projection-based imaging modalities relying upon measurements made at the target surface, reconstructed images are subject to noise in data acquisition and to artifacts due to the imaging algorithm and experimental conditions. The nature and magnitude of measurement errors must therefore be carefully factored in when trying to predict future clinical impacts of the new modalities and while prioritizing further technical improvements. This issue is important both when evaluating the clinical significance of a single image (where it may be appropriate to consider a range of possible images due to uncertainty in the measurements) and when developing summaries of many imaging sessions with respect to their diagnostic or prognostic value in the clinic. In this chapter, we describe efforts under way to develop statistical approaches for both single imaging studies and multimodality evaluation studies. Topics include confidence intervals for single images [1], techniques for summarizing the diagnostic value of images based on region-of-interest (ROI) summaries for single and multimodal studies [2], and empirical experiments on the character and magnitude of spatial accuracy across several imaging modalities [3].

2   STATISTICAL MODELING FOR SINGLE-IMAGE RECONSTRUCTION

2.1   Need for Statistical Methods

While x-ray computed tomography images can have a relatively well-defined image response with little apparent measurement error, model-based imaging methods may exhibit a complicated nonlinear relationship between measurement error and image accuracy. For example, in near infrared tomography, light propagation through tissue is modeled by diffusion theory and reconstructed images are derived by solution of the inverse problem [4, 5] (see Ch. 2 for discussion of the inverse problem and its converse, the forward problem). The inverse problem is typically ill-posed and ill-conditioned, requiring iterative optimization rather than exact solution. The derived images are generally of low resolution, although with proper calibration they may accurately reproduce average property values over specific areas of interest. Evaluation of reconstructed images requires consideration of statistical tools for assessment and visualization.

This chapter explores some possible analytical and graphical techniques for performing statistical inference on individual images. The concepts of statistical hypothesis testing and confidence are used to construct graphical presentations as aids for properly interpreting images known to contain noise. In particular, the concept of a "confidence interval" is extended as a means for visualizing the range of alternative images consistent with a particular set of sensor data. Techniques are illustrated with simulated images and phantom data from our alternative imaging program. Further details are available in [1] and [2].

2.2   Statistics of Finite Element Image Reconstruction

The finite element image reconstruction procedures used for image reconstruction in near infrared spectroscopic imaging (NIS), electrical impedance spectroscopy (EIS), magnetic resonance elastography (MRE), and microwave imaging spectroscopy (MIS) have many similarities [5–8]. All these procedures attempt to estimate the property distribution within a field representing the tissue, this field being discretized into a mesh of L nodal points. After the property values at these nodes are estimated, the resulting image estimate is constructed by interpolating values of individual pixels between adjacent nodes.

The reconstructed images specify a property coefficient $\theta(x_j, y_j)$ at each of $j = 1, \ldots J$ pixels. The interpolation process can be summarized by an equation relating the J pixel estimates to the L nodal points, i.e.,

$$\theta\left(x_j, y_j\right) = \sum_{\ell=1}^{L} \psi_\ell\left(x_j, y_j\right)\mu_\ell, \quad j = 1, \ldots J \tag{11.1}$$

where μ_ℓ represents the property value at the ℓth node and $\psi_\ell(x, y)$ represents a known interpolation or basis function (see Ch. 2). For our purposes, the number of pixels is assumed to be greater than the number of nodes (i.e., $J > L$).

Let $\mu = \{\mu_1, \mu_2, \ldots \mu_L\}^T$ denote an L-dimensional vector containing all of the node parameters. Further, let Φ_k^o, $k = 1, \ldots O_{IM}$ denote the signals from sensing devices at O_{IM} sites. These are the actual data available for constructing image estimates. It is reasonable to assume that each observed signal is a true signal (which is a function of the vector μ) plus a noise component:

$$\Phi_k^o = \Phi_k^c(\mu) + \varepsilon_k, \quad k = 1, \ldots O_{IM} \tag{11.2}$$

where each noise signal ε_k has zero mean and variance ϕ^2. The function $\Phi_k^c()$ is implicitly defined by partial differential equations (PDEs) specific to each imaging modality (as discussed further in the earlier chapters of this book). In the statistical literature, (11.2) might be referred to as a nonlinear regression model with parameters given by μ. Such models are the subject of an extensive theory of statistical analysis [4].

At the heart of the finite element image reconstruction is a least-squares problem in which an estimate $\hat{\mu} = \{\hat{\mu}_1, \hat{\mu}_2, \ldots \hat{\mu}_L\}^T$ of the property-parameter vector μ is obtained by minimizing the sum of squares with respect to μ, i.e., by minimizing

$$S(\mu) = \sum_{k=1}^{O_{IM}} \left(\Phi_k^o - \Phi_k(\hat{\mu}) \right)^2 \tag{11.3}$$

where $\Phi_k(\hat{\mu})$ is a predicted measurement based on the estimated parameter vector.

Direct optimization of (11.3) is difficult due to the multiplicity of parameters and the computational burden of numerically solving PDEs at each iteration of the least-squares optimization. Several approaches have been proposed to reduce these difficulties, including adaptive regularization of the Gauss-Newton method and spatial filtering [5]. More recent developments utilize statistical methods for ill-conditioned regression models to minimize bias due to the overspecified nature of the inverse problem [9, 10].

The theory of nonlinear least squares shows that under certain regularity conditions the parameter estimate $\hat{\mu}$ minimizing $S(\mu)$ converges to the true value of μ as the amount of data gets large (i.e., as $O_{IM} \to \infty$). This estimate will be asymptotically multivariate normal with a covariance matrix $\mathbf{M}$ that can be estimated as a by-product of the optimization procedure. However, estimation of $\mathbf{M}$ depends on the existence of a unique and stable solution for the optimization criterion. The corresponding theory for methods using regularization and other devices to improve the numerical algorithms is incomplete and does not provide variances for image estimates at this time. Below, some practical suggestions are discussed for obtaining variance estimates after procedures are described for performing statistical inferences that are possible once $\mathbf{M}$ has been estimated.

The image estimate can be represented as a J-dimensional vector $\hat{\theta}$ formed from the nodal parameters by substituting $\hat{\mu}$ in (11.1). Since these pixel estimates are simple linear functions of $\hat{\mu}$, the covariance matrix of the estimated image pixels is given by

$$\text{Cov}\left(\hat{\theta} \right) = \Psi \mathbf{M} \Psi^{\text{T}} \tag{11.4}$$

where Ψ is a $J \times L$ matrix with $\Psi_{j\ell} = \psi_\ell(x_j, y_j)$.

Using $\text{Cov}(\hat{\theta})$, we can provide analytic and graphical tools for assessing uncertainty about the properties of given areas within the image on a pixel-by-pixel basis. For instance, suppose that we wished to identify regions with optical property values greater than or less than a given level c. Because we can estimate the variance of each pixel as $\text{Cov}(\hat{\theta})_{jj}$, we can classify each pixel according to whether z is less than -1.96 or greater than 1.96, where

$$z = \frac{\hat{\theta}_j - c}{\sqrt{\text{Cov}(\hat{\theta})_{jj}}} \tag{11.5}$$

This is useful because viewing versions of the image which identify areas that are clearly different from a specified property value may help in locating abnormalities.

Statistical inference for entire images requires consideration of the extent to which pixel estimates are statistically correlated with one another. (This should be distinguished from the task of comparing individual pixels to a single reference level.) To judge the full range of possible images consistent with a reconstruction, one must consider the joint distribution of all pixel (or node) estimates. Simple confidence intervals for single means or other parameter estimates are commonly used in scientific reports; however, a simultaneous confidence interval for a highly dimensional estimate such as a reconstructed near infrared image takes the form of a confidence ellipse in the L dimensions of the node estimates $\hat{\mu}$. The true image then lies within the $(1 - \alpha)\%$ confidence ellipse with probability $(1 - \alpha)$, the "coverage probability" of the ellipse.

Visualization of these highly dimensional confidence ellipses poses a special graphical problem. One method is to show images on the surface of the ellipse corresponding to its widest principal axes. In effect, this gives a confidence interval for the most variable normalized linear combination of the pixel estimates. This method has been adopted using procedures involving orthogonal decompositions of the covariance matrix $\mathbf{M}$ (see [1]). The procedure can be repeated for the characteristic vectors corresponding to successively smaller characteristic values.

Figure 1 shows example images based on this procedure using a simulated image with an assumed value for $\mathbf{M}$ defined by a multiplicative error structure and an exponentially inverse relationship between pairwise pixel correlations and the distance separating pixels. By looking at these images, one can judge the range of reasonable images for the given sensor data. Note that the first pair of confidence-interval images (Image 1) weight the brighter of the two regions, since the multiplicative error structure means that these are also the most variable pixels. However, the brightest region is still detectable, looking at the lower-confidence-interval version of Image 1. The second pair of confidence-interval images (Image 2) primarily shows changes in

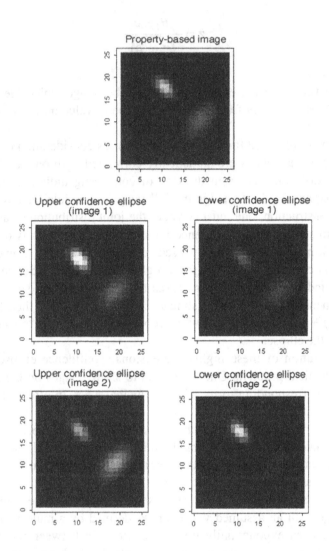

Figure 1. Confidence intervals for simulated images with multiplicative error structure and inter-pixel correlation decreasing with distance between pixels. Spatial units and grayscale are arbitrary for this synthetic data.

the larger region in the lower right quadrant. Given our assumptions about the variance of the pixel estimates in this area, the image corresponding to the lower limit of the confidence interval indicates that the data are consistent with an absence of the faint structure identified in the original image estimate.

These confidence-interval techniques require an estimate of $\mathbf{M}$. In theory, (11.3) can be used to develop suitable estimates. In practice, however, the choices for initial values, regularization parameters, and convergence criteria for the numerical optimization and PDE algorithms often result in unusable and potentially inaccurate values for $\mathbf{M}$, as defined by the gradient of the optimization criterion (11.3).

For the example given here, an alternative procedure has been adopted of dividing the signal measurement period into three equal segments and producing a triplicate set of node estimates from the three separate image reconstructions. These are used to empirically estimate the relationship between the distance separating two nodes and the correlation of their residuals from the node-specific means. An estimate of $\mathbf{M}$ is then formed by replacing the covariance term between any two nodes with the correlation predicted on the basis of the distance separating them multiplied by the square root of the product of the estimated variances at each node derived from the three replicate estimates.

Figure 2 shows the result of applying this procedure to a physical phantom with a single embedded object or anomaly imaged using our NIS technology. The true optical absorption image is computed from the known properties of the object and the relevant diffusion theory. Based on the three replicates, the average coefficient of variation for the absorption coefficient at each node is 1.4%. Because of a strong dependence of the residual variance on the mean, the node estimates were log-transformed prior to calculation of the covariance matrix for the image confidence intervals.

The confidence-interval images are plotted from the first two principal axes of the 95% confidence ellipse. Both statistical analyses indicate a region in the upper left quadrant with higher-than-average intensity. However, the intensity and exact location of the object are somewhat uncertain. A confidence map is also given in Figure 2 that shows elements of the image which differ from the overall mean with a statistical significance level of 5%, based on a two-sided t-test without any adjustments for multiple comparisons.

These graphical methods provide a means of guiding statistical inference for single images; other developments in the imaging literature have focused more on inferences for experimental designs comparing groups of images (see [11] for a summary of methods used in fMRI studies). The extension of the concepts of hypothesis testing and confidence intervals to imaging technology is not yet common, although there have been other treatments of uncertainty in imaging. Qi and Leahy [12], for example, present positron emission tomography voxel-specific variances in image format, where the variances are derived through the asymptotic theory of maximum likelihood estimation as applied to positron emission tomography image reconstruction. Their results for visualizing statistical tests and confidence intervals could also be applied in the setting of our program. However, for nonlinear image reconstruction applications, an empirical estimate of the covariance matrix for the estimated nodal parameters may be necessary. This is obtained by modifying data acquisition software to obtain replicate image reconstructions.

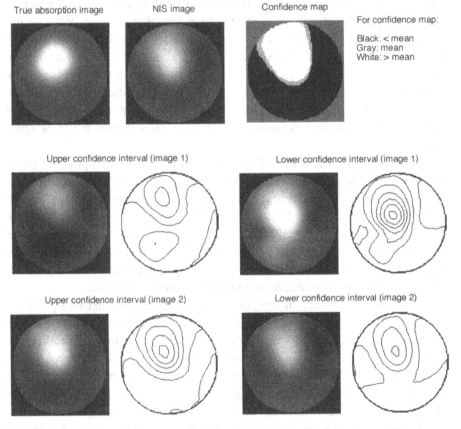

Figure 2. Confidence maps and confidence intervals for the absorption-coefficient image of a phantom with a single embedded object in the upper left quadrant. The true image is given in panel at upper left.

A key assumption in our methods is that image estimates are in fact unbiased, meaning that given an infinite number of replicated images the average reconstructed image will correspond precisely to the "true" image. Experimental projects described later in this chapter may help to provide empirical estimates of the potential for future improvements in these methods.

3   STATISTICAL METHODS FOR ASSESSING THE DIAGNOSTIC VALUE OF IMAGING

As part of our alternative imaging program, we are studying summary methods for diagnostic test variables derived from images. A clinical study currently in progress (2004) will compare imaging studies for 75 women having abnormal mammographic findings to those for 75 women having normal mammograms. All four modalities are included in this study. Image summaries will consist of average property values over entire images and within specific regions of interest, typically those marking the locations of possible abnormalities scheduled for biopsy. Statistical comparisons will focus on comparing the means of the property values of normal and abnormal tissues. The primary evaluation study is still in progress, but a preliminary study of normal subjects has been published [13] and some results are available for a limited number of abnormal patients.

Traditionally, diagnostic tests are characterized in terms of sensitivity (true-positive rate) and specificity (true-negative rate). With quantitative measures such as mean property values derived from images, the definition of test positivity involves specifying a cutoff beyond which a test result is considered abnormal. Receiver operating characteristic (ROC) curves plot sensitivity versus false-positive rate (1-specificity) as the cutoff is increased. For low values of the cutoff, fewer measurements from the abnormal group will test positive, while more from the normal group will test positive. There is an extensive literature on the use of ROC curves with either a continuous test variable or a categorized version of an underlying latent variable [14, 15]. The overall value of a diagnostic test is often summarized by the area under the ROC curve ("area under curve," AUC), which represents the probability that the test value for a normal subject exceeds that for an abnormal subject.

Two important issues arise in applying statistical methods for ROC curves to the data generated in the clinical evaluation studies from the Dartmouth program, namely (1) measurement error in the property values and (2) the use of test measures based on multiple imaging modalities. The topic of measurement error and ROC curves has generated recent interest in the statistical literature [16–19]. The primary finding from this work is that additional measurement errors will tend to move the ROC curve toward the "diagonal" line representing the ROC curve for a completely noninformative test and tend to reduce the AUC.

With our alternative breast imaging systems, it is possible to assess the accuracy of individual image summaries using the methods discussed in the previous section. Thus, each property mean over a specific region of interest has a corresponding standard error. Specialized statistical methods have been developed to take advantage of this information to create adjusted estimates of ROC curves [2]. Revised confidence bands and intervals for specific points on the binormal ROC curve have been developed to adjust for heteroscedastic and possibly non-normal measurement errors.

These methods can be described as follows. Let $d = 1$ indicate "abnormal" cases and $d = 0$ indicate "normal" cases. The true (unobserved) values for the test variable are denoted X_{di} for $i = 1,\ldots,n_d$ and $d = 0,1$ and are assumed to be normally distributed with mean μ_d and variance σ_d^2. The observed, error-prone values are denoted W_{di} for $i = 1,\ldots,n_d$ and $d = 0,1$ and are assumed to follow an additive measurement model, i.e.,

$$W_{di} = X_{di} + e_{di} \tag{11.9}$$

If $\tau_{di}^2 = \tau_d^2$ (constant variance within abnormal and normal groups), the sensitivity, specificity, and AUC based on W are given by

$$H(c) = 1 - \Phi\left(\frac{c - \mu_1}{\left(\sigma_1^2 + \tau_1^2\right)^{1/2}}\right), \quad 1 - P(c) = \Phi\left(\frac{c - \mu_0}{\left(\sigma_0^2 + \tau_0^2\right)^{1/2}}\right), \tag{11.11}$$

and

$$AUC = -\Phi\left(\frac{\mu_0 - \mu_1}{\left(\sigma_0^2 + \tau_0^2 + \sigma_1^2 + \tau_1^2\right)^{1/2}}\right) \tag{11.12}$$

Figure 3 shows the effect of increasing τ_0^2 and τ_1^2 on the ROC. Separate curves are shown for increasing values of the relative measurement error, $\kappa = (\tau_1^2 + \tau_0^2)/(\sigma_0^2 + \sigma_2^2)$. In general, an increase in measurement error moves the ROC curve towards the diagonal (noninformative) line and decreases the value of the AUC.

If there is measurement-error heterogeneity, the binormal model may not apply to the ROC based on W alone. This case is also illustrated in Figure 3, which shows examples where each observation is assigned its own separate measurement error variance (randomly generated to be lognormal and independent of X). The curves labeled a and b show the heterogeneous case with an average $\kappa = 1$ for a and $\kappa = 4$ for b. This example is analogous to what we expect for test data collected from the alternative imaging systems. Although the general effect of increasing measurement error is analogous to the homogenous case, the shapes of the ROC curves may be affected, and the heterogeneous case requires additional consideration in developing the estimation procedures.

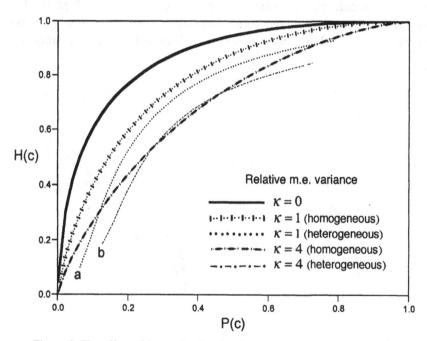

Figure 3. The effect of increasing levels of measurement error (m.e.) variance on ROC curves. Curves a and b show the effect of heterogeneous rather than homogeneous measurement-error variances.

Two possible methods have been explored for forming adjusted estimates and confidence intervals and confidence bands for ROC curves. The starting point for these methods is estimation of the mean and variance for each group, denoted by $\hat{\mu}_d$ and $\hat{\sigma}_d^2$ for group d. The first set of estimators consist of a simple unweighted mean and a method-of-moments estimate for $\hat{\sigma}_d^2$, i.e.,

$$\hat{\mu}_d = \tilde{W}_d \quad \text{and} \quad \hat{\sigma}_d^2 = s_{wd}^2 - \sum_i \hat{\tau}_{di}^2 \qquad (11.13)$$

These unweighted estimators are simple moment estimators and are always unbiased, even under heteroscedasticity. The second set of estimators is based on methods developed for meta-analysis [20] and incorporate the estimated measurement error variances as weighting factors. The meta-weighted estimates are of interest as a possible means of improving the efficiency of the estimated ROC curves.

The two methods are illustrated in Figure 4 using pathology data from the Dartmouth program [2]. For this example, vessel-density estimates and standard errors were obtained using automated image analysis with optical microscopy in specimens of normal and fibrocystic tissue. Results for unweighted and meta-weighted estimators are shown. Note how the corrected estimate of the ROC curve moves upwards away from the uncorrected

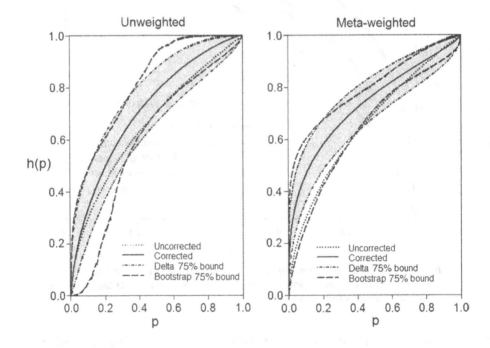

Figure 4. Example of an ROC curves corrected for heterogeneous measurement error and provided with 75% confidence bounds. Results for both weighted and meta-weighted estimators are shown.

curve (curve obtained when ignoring the presence of measurement error). This correlated estimate can be expected to be less biased than the uncorrected ROC curve. Confidence bounds are given for the corrected estimate using both an asymptotic (delta) approximation and a bootstrapping technique.

These results demonstrate that correction for measurement error in ROC curves is relatively simple and need not be limited to the AUC. However, more flexible assumptions about the distributions of the continuous test variables are needed [21], and the issue of the use of multiple imaging modalities needs to be addressed in this context. Preliminary data from our imaging program has provided an opportunity to consider methods for combining ROI measurements from multiple modalities. ROI analysis was performed for localized property enhancement relative to the background breast average for EIS, MIS, and NIS in 15 women subsequently found to have cancer. A comparable analysis was made of data from 8 women with benign conditions. In this study, the ROI was defined using a conventional mammogram.

Based on a simple comparison of means, the amount of localized property enhancement associated with cancer in all three modalities was encouraging. A multimodal index was formed using a linear discriminant function to optimally combine the three modalities. Figure 5 shows corresponding ROC curves plotted both empirically and as fitted binormal models with 95% confidence intervals. These preliminary results support a possible specificity

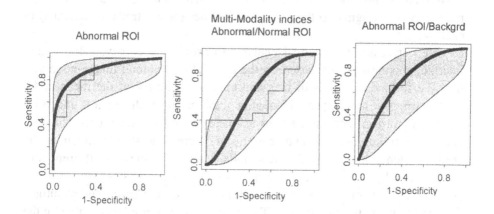

Figure 5. ROC curves and confidence intervals for three multimodality indices to discriminate cancer biopsies from non-cancer biopsies. The stairstep function represents the raw data; the heavy black line shows the ROC curve obtained by fitting a binormal model to the raw data. Shaded areas show 95% confidence intervals.

of approximately 80% with respect to pathologically benign lesions for a test based on the abnormal ROI multimodal index with a threshold small enough to detect 80% of cancers. This pretrial data are not subject to the same level of blinding and control as our evaluation trial (currently under way with mammographically normal and abnormal subjects), but nevertheless yield encouraging preliminary findings.

4   SPATIAL ACCURACY ACROSS IMAGING MODALITIES

To investigate the intermodal comparability and spatial accuracy in the early phase of technologies for EIS, NIS, and MIS, we performed an experiment with two sets of common phantoms that were repeatedly imaged by different modalities (EIS/NIS or MIS/NIS). This data has been reported in detail in [3] and is summarized here.

Each phantom was recorded in nine measurement sets in each imaging system: i.e., there were three separate sessions with three data acquisitions apiece. The sessions included a 10-minute electronics/optical system on/off interval, system recalibration, and phantom repositioning to simulate routine patient imaging sessions on different clinical days. To maintain identical positioning for all three modalities, each phantom was marked and carefully positioned within the detecting array of each imaging system, with the marker always aligned to the same optical fiber (or electrode, or antenna) in each system.

We performed a statistical analysis to estimate accuracy, validity, and intermodal comparability based on the data set of common image-node values. We formed estimates of bias and the standard error of the mean nodal value using the nine repeated imaging sessions for each imaging modality and phantom. Bias and standard-error images were formed for each phantom and modality combination and scatter plots were generated to illustrate the correspondence between individual nodal values obtained in different modalities. Finally, we computed the means of the bias and standard error images and used them in a two-way analysis of variance, treating the phantoms and modalities as the two factors. These analyses were used to summarize the comparisons of accuracy between the modalities.

Figure 6 gives spatial averages for the percentage bias and standard errors by imaging modality and type of phantom. Due to persistent artifacts at the image periphery in this set of experiments, the EIS shows a strong positive bias on the homogeneous and single-inclusion phantoms (top panel of

Fig. 6). All the modalities show a negative average bias on the phantoms with two inclusions, tending to smooth over these smaller features. The two-way analysis of variance of these data shows a statistically significant inter-modality comparison ($F = 5.81$, $p = 0.011$). The test for differences between phantoms is less significant ($F = 2.59$, $p = 0.09$).

The spatial averages for standard errors based on the repeated recon-structions are generally less than 10% (lower panel of Fig. 6). MIS, as ap-plied to the two-inclusion phantom, showed the highest standard error, 10.9%. The two-way analysis of variance of these data shows little evidence of a systematic difference according to phantom type ($R = 0.81$, $p = 0.54$) and only modest evidence of a difference between the modalities ($F = 2.28$, $p = 0.13$).

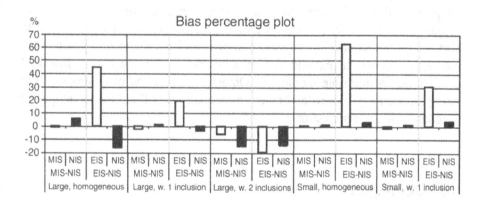

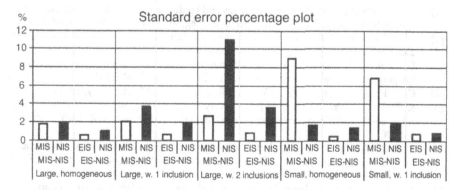

Figure 6. Percentage bias (top) and standard error (bottom) by imaging modality and phantom type.

Although average bias is shown in the analysis of variance to differ according to modality, strong spatial correlations are seen between individual images and between the percentage bias at each image node. Correlations between the bias at common nodes range from 0.68 for NIS and EIS applied to the small phantom with a single inclusion to 0.91 for NIS and MIS applied to the large phantom with a single inclusion. This suggests that the error structures for the imaging modalities are related, probably due to the use of a common image-reconstruction algorithm paradigm.

5   CONCLUSION

The statistical methods and experimental data described in this chapter attempt to deal with fundamental scientific and engineering issues in the development of multiple imaging modalities. Statistical methods are needed to portray the uncertainty in individual images and the diagnostic potential of image summaries in realistic clinical settings and for the comparison and combination of multiple modalities. Objective data-based evaluations of the scientific accuracy of new and emerging modalities will aid the development of reliable clinical applications.

REFERENCES

[1]   T. D. Tosteson et al., "Confidence maps and confidence intervals for near infrared images in breast cancer." *IEEE Trans. Med. Imaging*, Vol. 18(12), 1999, pp. 1188–1193.

[2]   T. D. Tosteson et al., "Measurement error and confidence intervals for ROC curves." *Biometrical Journal*, accepted with revision (2003).

[3]   D. Li et al., "Comparisons of three alternative breast modalities in a common phantom imaging experiment." *Medical Physics*, Vol. 30, 2003, pp. 2194–2205.

[4]   G. A. F. Seber and C. J. Wild, *Nonlinear Regression* (New York: Wiley, 1989).

[5]   K. D. Paulsen, and H. Jiang, "Spatially varying optical property reconstruction using a finite element diffusion equation approximation." *Med. Phys.*, Vol. 22(6), 1995, pp. 691–701.

[6]   K. D. Paulsen and H. Jiang, "Enhanced frequency-domain optical image reconstruction in tissues through total-variation minimization." *Appl. Opt.*, Vol. 35(19), 1996, pp. 3447–3458.

[7]   K. D. Paulsen and H. Jiang, "An enhanced electrical impedance imaging algorithm for hyperthermia applications." *Int. J. Hyperthermia*, Vol. 13(5), 1997, pp. 459–480.

[8]   J. T. Chang et al., "Non-invasive thermal assessment of tissue phantoms using an active near field microwave imaging technique." *Int. J. Hyperthermia*, Vol. 14(6), 1998, pp. 513–534.

[9]   P. M. Meaney et al., "A two-stage microwave image reconstruction procedure for improved internal feature extraction." *Med. Phys.*, Vol. 28(11), 2001, pp. 2358–2369.

[10] E. Demidenko, *Modeling Longitudinal and Spatially Correlated Data* (New York: Springer-Verlag, 1997), pp. 47–62.

[11] N. Lange, "Statistical approaches to human brain mapping by functional magnetic resonance imaging." *Stat. Med.*, Vol. 15(4), 1996, pp. 389–428.

[12] J. Qi and R. M. Leahy, "A theoretical study of the contrast recovery and variance of MAP reconstructions from PET data." *IEEE Trans. Med. Imag.*, Vol. 18(4), 1999, pp. 293–305.

[13] P. P. Poplack et al., "Electromagnetic breast imaging—average tissue property values in normal women." *Radiology*, Vol. 231, 2004, pp. 571–580.

[14] J. Hanley, "ROC curves." In *Encyclopedia of Biostatistics*, P. Armitage and T. Colton, eds. (London: Wiley, 1998).

[15] C. B. Begg, "Advances in statistical methodology for diagnostic medicine in the 1980s." *Stat. Med.*, Vol. 10, 1991, pp. 1887–1895.

[16] M. Coffi and S. Sukhatme, "Receiver operating characteristic studies and measurement errors, *Biometrics*, Vol. 53, 1997, pp. 823–837.

[17] D. Faraggi, "The effect of measurement error on ROC curves." *Stat. Med.*, Vol. 19, 2000, pp. 61–70.

[18] B. Reiser, "Measuring the effectiveness of diagnostic markers in the presence of measurement error through the use of ROC curves." *Stat. Med.*, Vol. 19, 2000, pp. 2115–2129.

[19] E. F. Schisterman et al., "Statistical inference for the area under the receiver operating characteristic curve in the presence of measurement error." *American Journal of Epidemiology*, Vol. 154, 2001, pp. 174–179.

[20] B. J. Biggerstaff and R. L. Tweedie, "Incorporating variability in estimates of heterogeneity in the random effects model in meta-analysis." *Stat. Med.*, Vol. 16, 1997, pp. 753–768.

[21] K. H. Zou, W. J. Hall, and D. E. Shapiro, "Smooth non-parametric receiver operating characteristic (ROC) curves for continuous diagnostic tests." *Stat. Med.*, Vol. 16, 1997, pp. 2143–2156.

INDEX

A
absorption (in NIS), 9, 193–194, 194f, 213–217, 217f
adipose tissue. See breast, anatomy of
adjoint method of calculating Jacobian, 38–40, 92–93
Agilent synthesized RF source, 157–159, 160f, 164
antenna selection (in MIS), 137–138
area under curve, 235–240

B
β dispersion, 6
banded matrix, 28
basis function(s), Lagrangian, 28–33, 30f, 31f, 36–37, 53, 147
Bayesian statistics, 64–66
Beowulf cluster, 60, 60f
Boltzmann equation, 202
boundary conditions, 33
    EIS, 33, 88–89
    MIS, 33, 132–137, 133f, 139–144, 140f, 142f
    MRE, 33
    NIS, 33, 184, 187–188, 197
boundary element(s), 33, 132–137, 133f, 140f
breast(s)
    anatomy of, 10, 169f, 220
    cancer of. See cancer, breast
    electrical properties of, 6, 7–8, 128, 169–172, 171f, 172f
    electromechanical properties of, 5, 17, 18f, 18t, 19t, 69, 79–82, 80f–82f
    interface with in EIS, 7, 88–89, 93, 112 –113, 118f
    interface with in MIS, 7, 166–168, 167f
    interface with in MRE, 72–73, 72f, 73f, 74f, 76, 77f
    interface with in NIS, 8, 204–214, 209f
    isotropy of, 88
    optical properties of, 9, 17, 18f, 18t, 19t, 213–220, 214f, 215f, 217f–219f
    physiology of, 10–20, 13f, 169, 238–239, 238f, 239f
    radiologically dense, 3, 178–180, 179f, 180f
    radiologically scattered, 171–172, 171f, 172f

C

cancer, breast. See also fibroadenoma; malignant neoplasm
    ductal, 216, 217f, 218f, 219f
    electrical properties of, 8, 86, 86f
    infiltrating ductal, 16
    mechanical properties of, 69–70
    optical properties of, 9
    physiology of, 10–20, 15f
    prevalence of, 1
    tissue morphology of, 9–20
CD31 stain, 12, 13f, 15f, 20
chromophores, 214–216
clinical breast exam, 1–2
clinical core, 4, 20–21, 21f
coarse mesh. See property mesh
complete electrode model, 89
computational
    core, 4, 20–21, 21f
    efficiency, 36, 38, 40, 55–58, 63, 64f
condition number of Jacobian, 41
confidence intervals for images, 230–233, 232f
confidence map, of NIS absorption image, 233–234, 234f
conformal mesh approach, 149–150, 150f
continuum model, 89
contrast-to-noise ratio, 78
correlation
    cross-modality, 17, 19t, 240–242, 241f
    Spearman, 12–13
cost function, 34
covariance matrix, 230–234
CT. See x-ray computed tomography
cytokeratin 5D3, 14f

D

deoxyhemoglobin, 206, 213, 216
detectability of low-contrast lesions, 76–79, 79f–82f
diagnostic value, statistical assessment of, 235–240
diffusion equation, 27, 184–187, 203
digital signal processing chips, 117–122, 120f
direct method of calculating Jacobian, 92
Dirichlet boundary condition, 140

G

Galerkin method, 31–32
gap model, 89
Gauss-Newton method, 26, 33–35, 130–137, 155
geometries, imaging, 204–206, 204f
glandular tissue. See breast, anatomy of
global property value estimation, 98, 99f
glycerin, 166–168, 168f
Green's
    function, 133–134, 141–144, 142
    identity, 32, 37

H

hardware design process, goals of, 155–157
Helmholtz equation, 26–27, 37, 132
hematoxylin and eosin stain, 11–12
hemoglobin concentration (Hb_T), 10–11, 17, 18t, 206, 213–214, 214f, 215f
Hessian matrix, 43–44, 131, 146
Hooke's Law, 27, 51
hybrid element(s)
    forward solution, 132–136, 133f
    in nonactive antenna compensation, 139–144, 140f, 142f
    reconstruction, 136–137

I

ill-conditioning, of inverse problem, 41–45, 228
illumination tank. See microwave imaging spectroscopy, breast interface
intercapillary distance, 19
inverse problem, 25, 33–41
    ill-conditioning of, 41–45
    in MIS, 135–137
    in NIS, 189–193
    with hybrid elements, 136–137
iteration step size, 45
iterative solutions, 28

J

Jacobian matrix, 35, 38–40, 41, 53, 55, 91–93, 136, 147–148, 189–190, 190f

L

Lagrangian basis function. See basis function(s), Lagrangian